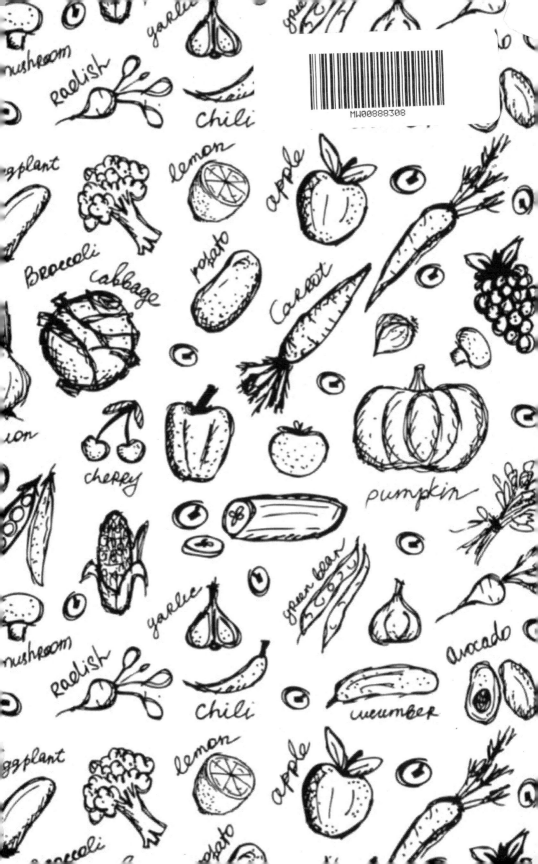

Clean Eating With Kids
Carey Wood
First Edition © 2014 Carey Wood

www.cleaneatingwithkids.com

DISCLAIMER

The Author is not a Nutritionist or a Doctor. The information in this book is provided for information purposes only. If you have any allergies or concerns about your health, please consult your general practitioner.

Clean Eating with Kids

A Real Family's Guide on How to Eat Clean when you have kids, work, school lunches, busy days and a real life.

CAREY WOOD

ACKNOWLEDGMENTS

This book is for all you fearless Parents who have chosen to clean up your family's diet. You know it's going to rock that sometimes tender balance in your household and you are pretty sure everyone isn't going to be 'ecstatic' with your decision, but – You're doing it anyway!

I already know that we are kindred spirits. I hope that our kids sit together in the school lunchroom so that when they glance across at each other's lunch boxes, they get to see that they are not the only ones with a crazy Mom or Dad who loves them enough to say 'No' to the crap.

Thank you for joining me on this Journey.

"We have to dare to be ourselves, however frightening or strange that self may prove to be."

— May Sarton

CONTENTS

REAL LIFE

Real life happens. There will be birthday parties, Easter egg hunts, school functions and plenty of special occasions that will rock your clean eating boat. Life loves to present little challenges, but as parents, we work through them. It's all part of the job.

Before you jump into your new clean eating lifestyle, please remember, everyone is different. Do what works for your family. Don't be too hard on yourself or your kids. Many of you will be making some big changes to your family's diet. Whether it's a couple of easy tweaks or a major diet overhaul - Remember - any positive change you make, big or small, is a step in the right direction.

With love.
Carey,
Busy Mum to 4 gorgeous kids (who aren't always on the same Clean Eating page as me).

PART 1

GETTING STARTED

ABOUT THIS BOOK

The food that we are feeding our kids is not OK. It's pretty obvious that something is seriously wrong with our food supply. What we eat is making us (and our kids) fat and sick; and we are too damn busy to put up a fight.

I get it. Family life *is busy*. We juggle all day to keep it together, and then still do our best to get home and cook up a healthy dinner from scratch, clean up, go to bed and do it all again the next day. When we don't get this right, that's when the guilt sets in ...

As parents, we want the best for our children. Our simple wish is for them to grow up healthy and happy. For me, this included teaching my children to eat real food and to set a good example for them to follow. This is our family's story on how we began to clean up our eating habits - in spite of real life.

I have broken the book into two parts. Part 1 deals with the nitty grittys of what we did to change our bad eating habits and make the move to clean eating. Don't be put off by the process. We are all creatures of habit. Once something becomes a habit, it doesn't require much effort to keep it going. Clean Eating is no different.

Part 2 is packed full of Clean Eating Recipes. I'm not a photographer or a chef. You won't find glossy pictures or complicated recipes. There are only real-life, family friendly dishes that I cook regularly for my kids. I know most of them by heart and can put the majority of the meals together faster than the time it would take me to go get a takeaway. Best of all, - ALL of the ingredients used in my recipes can be sourced easily from your local Supermarket or farmers market no matter where you are in the World.

"If you don't know where you're going, any road'll take you there"

— George Harrison

IT'S TIME TO ROCK THE BOAT

So you've decided to start eating clean but you don't know where to start? Oh Baby, have we been there! If you've picked up this book, I can assume that you are unhappy with the food you are feeding your family and are looking for an answer on how to make the change to a healthier lifestyle without total anarchy in your home.

This book started as a scrappy recipe binder in my kitchen. It's full of practical ideas and simple recipes that helped our family on our road to eating real food. I am not a chef or a nutritionist. I am just a Mother who needed to drastically rethink the food I was feeding my family.

A couple of promises I will make about the contents and recipes in this book:

1. There are no complicated recipes or hard to find ingredients. As lovely as Agave Nectar and coconut sugar are, they just don't feature in this book.

2. Our household operates on a tight budget. All of the recipes are budget friendly and designed to help you eat whole foods on a realistic budget.

3. We are a real life family with the same real life issues that you have. Life is busy. There's work, school pickups, after school sports, sometimes sick kids, homework emergencies and countless last minute melodramas. Like you, I still want to feed my family healthy food and get it on the table fast – every single day!

4. You are not alone. Thousands of parents wake up every day with the same nagging feeling that something is not right with our food system. Don't feel the pressure to give in and settle for anything less. Protect yourself and your family by choosing to eat clean, real foods.

Eating clean is a no brainer. You are feeding your family fresh, real whole foods and staying away from the processed, plastic stuff. Sound simple? Huh!

The reality is - many of us have slipped very far down the processed food rabbit hole. We've been sold the line "better, bigger, vitamin enriched & good for your kids" and we fell for it. We live our lives on the run. 50 years ago only 12% of mothers worked full time, now that figure is close to 60%.

Time is our Number 1. priority and we vote with our dollar by purchasing pre-made, preservative full foods that we can feed our kids – fast. Marketing surveys show that around a third of most household's food budgets are spent on prepared foods away from the home. We treat our kids by taking them to the local fast food drive through and we feel guilty when our children take a lunch box to school holding 'just' a sandwich and some fruit.

The lifestyle of the modern family has shifted. It has been designed to serve an ever profitable food industry. The result is that our children's health is suffering and we are not even putting up a fight.

"We may not be able to prepare the future for our children, but we can at least prepare our children for the future."

— Franklin D. Roosevelt

CLEAN EATING IN A NUTSHELL

Supermarkets popped up on the scene in the early 1900's. Since then the race was on to stock their shelves with the cheapest, nastiest, profit generating products possible. Our children are being raised thinking that milk is made in a factory and fruit comes in pretty plastic wrappers – with added sugar and no seeds! Never before has food been so available.

Back in 1930, renowned economist John Keynes predicted that technological advancements would mean we would all eventually work just 15 hours a week. And yet, according to the Gallop 2014 Work and Education survey, the old "9 to 5" work week is becoming obsolete. Economically-stressed Americans are now working an "average" of 47 hours, with a growing number clocking 60 hours or more.

Adults employed full time in the U.S. report working an average full workday longer than what a standard five-day 9-to-5 schedule. As a result, time spent in the kitchen preparing food from scratch has taken a dive.

We are constantly under pressure to do things faster. Families operate on a tight schedule to fit everything in. We have been sold the line that meal preparation is a 'hassle' that takes up 'too much time', why not drive to the nearest drive through or grab breakfast 'on the go'. Time saving technology is everywhere, yet we feel rushed.

Our society is now seeing the dramatic effect of this lifestyle. Our health is suffering, obesity rates are souring and the link between real food and the stuff we are eating is getting blurred. We need to find a way to safeguard our family's health despite modern living.

Technology is here to stay and a long work hour week is a reality to many. Most parents do not have the time to spend hours in the kitchen preparing food like our grandmothers did a couple generations ago, but despite this, we still have to accept responsibility for the food we feed our family. For us, clean eating is the solution.

Clean Eating has been around a long, long time.

The goal of Clean Eating is to simply eat simple food in their most natural, nutritionally dense state, or as close to it as possible. It's not a new idea or 'latest diet'. It's just the way we are meant to eat. Somewhere in the past three generations, we lost our way.

So, What Exactly is Clean Eating?

- It's about eating whole foods as close to their natural state as possible. Food that exists naturally like meat and poultry, eggs, whole grains, fish, beans and legumes, vegetables, fruit, nuts and seeds and dairy.
- It is a lifestyle of choosing real food over processed food.
- It's about improving the quality of the food you feed your family.
- It's about being in control of your health.
- It's knowing and caring about where your food comes from.

- It's about living the life you were meant to live.
- Teaching your kids to make good food choices.
- Feeding your family healthy, nutrient rich foods.
- Eating good food, more often.
- It's about teaching our children to recognize the BS fed to them every day in the form of marketing messages, advertising and the media.

What Clean Eating is NOT.

- It is not complicated.
- It doesn't require you to count calories or weigh your food.
- It is not a diet.
- It is not new.
- It's not an endless list of 'revolutionary' new super foods that you have never heard of and now 'can't live without'.
- It's not low-fat, low-cholesterol, vegetarian or vegan.
- It's not boring or tasteless.

"Any food that requires enhancing by the use of chemical substances should in no way be considered a food."

— John H. Tobe

WHY DO IT? WHY EAT CLEAN IN THE FIRST PLACE?

The Signs are everywhere that something is wrong with our food industry. What we are feeding our kids is now a very real problem.

According to Michael Pollan[1], author of An Omnivores Dilemma, many chronic diseases can be traced back to the industrialization of our food, including diabetes and cancer. It's a global problem and our children are suffering the effects of our choices. It is more important, than ever before, that we teach our children how to eat for their health.

There will be days that the decision to eat clean just seems too hard. You need to focus on the reasons that you are making these changes. Find your *Reason Why*. Remind yourself why it's important to you that your family eats real food.

Eating Clean has changed how our family thinks of food. I want to teach my children to be aware of, and accountable for, the food they eat. My goal is for them to grow to be healthy adults who care about the World around them.

For our family, the obvious effects from a couple of weeks Clean Eating were:

1. My children were generally happier, calmer and balanced.
2. They started sleeping well,
3. They were hungry at the right times and
4. We all had more energy.
5. Both my big kids complexions became clearer within a couple of days.
6. Everyone went to the toilet regularly (I know, a bit of a icky subject, but I needed to get it out there).
7. And to top it, I feel more confident in my abilities as a Mother.
8. We are now aware of exactly where our food is coming from - from locally sourced vegetables to how our meat came to be on our plates. These were subjects I just hadn't bought up before. So much so that my 5yr old once asked "What's chicken made of?" A very interesting discussion followed.

Basic health benefits of eating clean, whole foods include:

- Improved immunity
- Weight management
- Clearer Complexion
- Increased energy
- Regular Bowel Function
- Children enjoying a healthy diet are more likely to grow into adults who do the same.

Changing towards a clean eating diet may feel a bit overwhelming at first, especially if you have a lot of changes to make. Don't over think it. Your goal is to prepare good, fresh foods that will keep your family healthy.

Whether you are aiming for 100% clean eating lifestyle, or if you just want to supplement a meal a day. It's is up to you. Do what works for your family.

"No disease that can be treated by diet should be

treated with any other means."

— Maimonides

THE FAT FACTS: ARE YOU MAKING YOUR CHILD FAT?

When the effects of a bad diet are hidden, it's easy to ignore. But one of the more visible effects of our sugar enriched, added fat and highly processed lifestyle is now becoming very hard to ignore. Our kids are getting fatter.

No parent likes to admit that their child is overweight. And yet, obesity is one of the most common health conditions amongst modern children and teenagers. In 2012 more than one third of children and adolescents in developed nations were overweight or obese. In the US alone, the obesity rate has tripled over the past 30 years. Tripled! More than 23 million kids and teenagers are now obese or overweight.

From 1980 – 2012, the number of US children aged 6-11 years who were considered obese increased from 7% to 18%. Adolescent obesity rates increased from 5% to 21% in that same time.

These numbers aren't restricted to the US. Australia, Europe and now China are seeing similar statistics. As technology and industry soars, so does our children's weight.

The early human race adapted to living in a world of scarcity. We ate when we could in order to survive. We naturally developed a taste for sweet, fatty foods that could provide us with energy to survive. Overabundance was not an issue.

Our bodies were designed to conserve energy for periods when we needed it – to hunt or defend ourselves. In other words, our bodies are really good at putting on weight and it works hard to keep it there. If you have ever been on a diet, you will know exactly what I am talking about here.

We are naturally attracted to sweet, high energy foods and food industry manufacturers are well aware of this. We are not equipped to deal with an abundant supply of energy rich foods available to us so we have to learn to manage the food we put into our system. We can no longer blame food industry manufacturers or point fingers. We are aware of the faults in the system and it is now our responsibility to educate ourselves and manage the food we allow into our homes.

I'm not going to lie to you. Chocolate, sugar donuts and fried chicken burgers appeal to our taste buds. We love the taste of processed foods and so do our kids. Our bodies are designed that way. And that is what makes it so very scary. Time and time again it's been shown that diets fail because people feel as if they are being deprived of the 'good stuff'. As soon as the diet ends, we rush for the closest donut shop. Tad dramatic, but you get the idea.

You have heard this before – and I am going to say it again – The *only way* you can get your family to adopt a Clean Eating lifestyle is to accept that it is a lifestyle and not a diet. As parents, our goals are to teach and empower our children with knowledge. Once they reach adulthood, they will be free to make their own choices. We just have to hope that they choose wisely. Children that grow up seeing their parents make healthy eating choices, are more inclined to do the same when they reach adulthood.

"Everything depends on upbringing. "

— Leo Tolstoy, War and Peace

IS IT CLEAN? THE 4 STEP TEST

When you start making the move from processed to whole food living, you can easily become obsessed with letters, numbers, chemical food names etc. I was overwhelmed by the details and I nearly gave up. I thought it all too hard. For some reason, I had it in my head that this was a pass or fail affair and that I was a failure if I misread a label or found that the orange juice my kids had drunk for breakfast was 'vitamin enriched'.

So, to keep it simple, here are 4 Questions to ask before choosing whether or not to add it to your shopping basket or dinner plate:

1. **Do you know what that ingredient is?** In all of my 37years (and travels), I figure I have come across many a food type. If I don't know what it is yet, or if I don't recognize it as food or if I need to look it up, or if it comes with a number at the end, then I am pretty sure we can survive without it.

   For those of you who are a bit more adventurous than me, there is an amazing App called "Chemical Maze". Download it onto your phone and you can instantly look up any ingredient. I think they even produce a little soft cover reference book for the unsavvy techies out there.

2. **Did it grow or was it made?** You don't see bags of Cheezels growing in neat rows in your garden. Choose real, whole foods that are closest to their natural state as possible. The less processed the better.

3. **How far did it travel to get here?** Choose local wherever you can. Shopping at your local farmers markets or green grocer is not just about getting fresh, seasonal produce.

4. **Was it humanly produced?** The Food Industry is big business and we are its customers. Use your Shopping dollars to make a difference by choosing foods that are sustainable and humanely produced. 'Vote' with your dollar by purchasing goods produced by companies that care for our world.

"I mean, when the world comes for your children, with the knives out, it's your job to stand in the way."

— Joe Hill, Horns

OUR LIFE BEFORE CLEAN EATING

Before we started eating clean, our family ate like a lot of other busy families. Meals were chosen for how quickly I could get them on the table, and whether or not it would be easy to get my kids to actually eat it. Fast and fuss free, baby. We ate many a meal in the car on the way to places. I wasn't consciously aware of how few fruits and vegetables my children were eating and I didn't even consider what was actually in the food I handed over from the front seat of my car.

It wasn't always like that.

When I had my first child, I started off with the very best of intentions. Baby #1 was blessed with home cooked meals and real food made with love – for the first year of her life. When baby #2 arrived 15 months later, I started buying the odd bottled baby food "to get me through" the busy evenings. I struggled with juggling a new baby, hungry toddler and building our business.

Then baby #3 and #4. Most evenings I was making two separate meals. If I were really honest, sometimes I prepared three meals – one for parents, one for big kids and one for little kids. Sounds Crazy? I know. I just wanted my kids to eat food without a fight, so I pretty much served them what they wanted. I was creating my very own pack of little monsters.

Going out to dinner at friends and family was always a bit stressful. My children weren't used to eating what was on their plate. I often made excuses as to why my children weren't eating the food in front of them. I dreaded hearing them say, "I don't like this". I was embarrassed and would make excuses like, "Oh, they are feeling a bit sick", or "She had a big lunch". I also knew that that same child would happily have munched down it's body weight in donuts if they were available. Sometimes I would bet home from dinner with hungry kids and full them up on toast. It was ridiculous.

Around the time my youngest son turned 5, I discovered the virtues of Clean Eating almost by mistake. I felt tired all the time and I was unhappy in my own body. I started eating clean to lose weight. In the beginning it was 'just another diet'. It didn't even cross my mind to change my family's diet too.

I had been eating clean for about a week. I was losing weight, felt really great – and all was good, until, one night I looked up from my plate of fresh chicken and veggie stir-fry. My dining table was full of old papers, a massive pile of washing waiting to be folded and a bowl of less than edible fruit.

My children were lined up on the couch eating their beige colored food that I had lovingly defrosted and heated up in the oven. No one took their eyes off the TV screen. It hit me. I should have been doing better. Why wasn't I? I know what real food is, why wasn't I feeding it to my kids? When do you wake up and start to make changes? When someone gets sick? Maybe no one get sick. Maybe. That night we started eating clean (with 4 'not-so-happy-with-the-idea' kids and a very skeptical husband).

Up until that moment, if you had asked me, I would have said that we ate OK. I actually thought that we didn't eat too badly. I mean, there was SOME chicken in those frozen chicken nuggets and surely there was SOME potato in those oven fries. I always had fruit in the house (most days in the form of fruit juice) but normally a couple of sad looking apples at the back of the fridge.

School lunches were another problem I encountered the very next morning. For years, I think have been putting the same apple back into my children's lunch boxes every day. They never ate it, and I just kept recycling it. Hmmm. Mommy of the year award right there; and a high five for that amazing, never aging apple.

Then there is the issue of Peer Pressure. Oh wow. That never goes away. You get to experience it all over again when your children start day care, kindergarten or school.

Peer Pressure at school often influences the contents of the lunch box. Whatever "Everyone Else" has in their lunch box starts to dictate what you buy at the Store. Television adverts and pretty packaging make it all that bit harder - the Food Industry spends a sordid amount of money telling our kids what food they should eat – Peer Pressure.

Our family had so many bad habits in place. The decision to make the change to clean eating required a major overhaul of our diet.

In the beginning, these were the 10 basic steps I our family took to begin Clean Eating:

1. Clean out our pantry & fridge & get rid of all processed foods in our home.
2. Drink Water. No More Soda, Fruit Juice or Cordial.
3. Make sure everyone gets their 5 a day of fruit and veg.
4. Plan and shop for 1 week of Clean Meals including snacks and school lunches.
5. Always have TWO emergency meals available (A frozen serve of Bolognaise sauce and chicken stew worked well for me).
6. Everyone eats the same meal. No more cooking variations to suit fussy eaters or to try and please everyone.

7. Clear my dining room table and eat dinner together at least three times a week. I had to keep reminding myself that the Dining Table was for food, not washing.
8. Add one new meal a week to my recipe book (yes you are now holding that recipe book)
9. Simplify School lunches – one sandwich (on whole grain), one fruit, one veg and one homemade snack.
10. Taught my children about how to assess whether a food is clean. This was easier than I thought it would be. Kids love rules, so this became a bit of a game (and the four step test was invented (see pg 24)

Clean Eating is definitely a process.

Think of it as introducing good food into your home that will slowly replace or push out the bad stuff.

So for example:

1. Replace Soda with Water

2. Replace White Bread with Wholemeal

3. Replace Snack Bars with Homemade granola bars

4. Replace processed snacks with fruit or popcorn

5. Remake meals using clean ingredients

"Wolves Don't Lose Sleep Over The Opinions Of Sheep."

Unknown

A WORD ON MODERATION AND SHEEP.

Once you start making changes in your life, the people around you will put up resistance. To varying degrees, you will be judged, you may be criticized and you will, most definitely, doubt your decisions.

This is your life. You only get one. And the older I get, the more I realize that we are all making up the Rules as we go. Decide on your Rules and do what works for you and your family.

10 THINGS WE DID WHEN WE STARTED EATING CLEAN

(WITH 4 NOT-TOO-HAPPY KIDS AND 1 NOT ON THE SAME PAGE HUSBAND)

TIP # 1
Overhauling your pantry and fridge

When you decide to start your clean eating lifestyle, one of the first things you will need to do is to clear your kitchen of all processed foods. Now there are two ways of doing this:

1. Use up what is in your pantry and gradually introduce real food, whilst using up what you have. OR you can ...

2. Go Cold Turkey. Clean out your pantry all in one go. If it's not real food, then dump it or donate it. My theory is this: if it's not in your house, then you can't eat it. This is the route I chose, but I must warn you that you need to be prepared. Have food in the cupboards and meal plans ready to go. I tossed out all the crap, but ended up with an empty pantry and hungry kids.

As a parent, you are in control of the food you make available to them by keeping it in your cupboard. Self Control is a Myth. PLAN AHEAD! Don't keep food in the house that you don't want your kids to eat.

If a decision making member of your family isn't totally on board, (Ahem ... like my husband), then allocate them a spot in out of sight cupboard to keep their stash. It avoids any issues with children wanting what you don't want them to eat. Don't make it difficult for yourself.

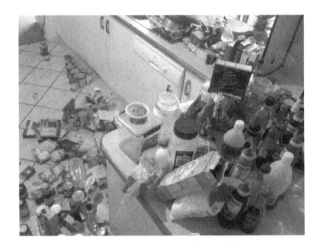

The Day I cleaned out our Pantry. The only thing I kept was the little pile of cans in the far back of the picture!

Remove all refined, packaged foods.

Bag it all up, take it to a food bank or homeless shelter. The kids do NOT need potato chips, sugary biscuits or salted crackers available in your home. Trust me; they will have sufficient access to them outside of your home – school, friend's houses, parties etc. Keep it out of your home.

Prepping your Pantry

A well stocked pantry makes life so much easier. Obviously, the contents of your pantry are limited by your family's budget; however, keeping your pantry stocked with a few basics will save you money and stop you splurging on last minute meals. Try to stock your pantry slowly with ingredients that you can use to make a few meals from scratch.

Keep your Pantry stocked with clean, whole foods like:

- Minimally processed foods – whole wheat flour, canned beans and lentils, canned tomatoes, maple syrup, frozen vegetables, canned tuna and salmon, canned water packed fruits, organic dried fruits, organic peanut butter, unsweetened apple sauce, organic pasta sauce.
- Whole grains – whole grain Pasta, Whole grain Rice, Rye Bread, 100% whole grain cereals and oats, whole grain wraps or tortillas
- Natural Salad Dressings
- Brown Rice Cakes
- 100% wholegrain crackers
- Raw and unprocessed foods – brown rice, nuts and seeds, honey and dried beans, garlic, potatoes and onions; popcorn seeds.
- Preservative free – oils, vinegar, herbs and spices, sea salt

The move towards conscious eating is growing. Supermarkets are responding to demand by stocking a wider range of minimally processed, natural food products that would easily fit within your clean lifestyle.

NOTE: In Part 2 of this book, I have done my best to use simple ingredients in all of my recipes. I have chosen not to include the wide range of options available as availability may vary depending on where you live and your budget. I have tried to include ingredients that would be available to most households.

Clean Foods that I keep in my fridge:

- Organic butter, cottage cheese, sour cream, milk, almond milk, cheeses and Greek yogurt.
- Free range eggs
- Free range meats and fish
- Condiments – Clean salad dressing, organic ketchup, chutney, mayonnaise and jams. (yes, you can make these, but there are plenty of good options available at most supermarkets).
- Homemade fruit juices
- Fresh fruits, lettuce, vegetables, fresh herbs
- Dips: Hummus, salsa
- Leftover meat slices – roast chicken, roast beef etc

Inside a Well Stocked Freezer :

- Frozen fruits and vegetables
- Fish and Meats
- Homemade treats – fruit pops, ice cream
- Homemade meals – Pasta Sauce, Soups, Chicken or Vegetable Stock.
- Organic, 100% whole wheat sliced bread

I try to stock about a week's worth of meals in my freezer. More than that seems to get wasted and starts to take up needed space. See the references at the back of this book for a clean food shopping list.

TIP #2
Leave the kids at home.

The Supermarket is not your friend. It is designed to work against you. The Big Chain Marketers work really hard to encourage those last minute' purchases i.e. the chocolate or cold soda drink you add to the basket when standing in line to pay.

Add a child to the mix and they have their very own personal shopper following you around the store. It takes a strong parent to say No every time. I have seen many a Mom cave at this point in the clean shopping cycle – myself included.

When you start eating clean, I would advise making that first supermarket trip on your own. Take your time to browse the aisles. You will need to look at it all with new eyes.

TIP #3
Plan Your Go to meals (Because you WILL need them)

Plan three quick and easy meals that will work as your 'Go to meals'. These are the meals that you can get on the table in 10-15 minutes flat (as long as it's less time than it would take to drive to the closest takeaway outlet).

Make sure that you always have ingredients on hand to make these – ALWAYS!!! Some good examples are: -

- Eggs – Scrambled, boiled served with Rye Toast and carrot sticks

- Frozen bolognaise sauce (just defrost and stir through wholemeal pasta and add your choice of frozen veg)

- Frozen soups (defrost and serve with toasted Rye). I keep 100% whole wheat or rye bread in my freezer at all times.

- Quiche – add frozen or thinly sliced fresh vegetables, egg and cheese. Serve with a side of salad for a quick, yummy dinner or lunch.

Visit **www.cleaneatingwithkids.com** for more clean eating, kid friendly recipes.

TIP #4
Read the ingredients.

If you don't know what's in it, don't put it in your shopping basket. You do not need a degree in nutrition at this point. Start simple. Start with what you know.

Try not to purchase foods that have more than 3-6 ingredients in the ingredient list. And be sure you recognize each and every ingredient listed. As you get used to Clean Eating your knowledge on this will grow naturally. Remember to check it before you eat it. Do the research once and add it to your shopping list for good.

The Secret to buying bread (Is it really as sinful as everyone makes out?)

Our family loves bread. It forms a good part of our diet - from morning toast to lunchtime sandwiches. I know that it is not very fashionable right now to admit this, but we eat bread daily. Like most things in life, not all bread is bad, and not all bread is created equal.

Before Clean Eating, we would delight in thick sliced, highly processed white bread. It was what we identified as 'bread'. Changing to clean, wholegrain bread was one of the bigger adjustments we had to make in our new lifestyle. In the beginning, two of my children were not happy with the bread change in our home, so I did a couple of things to fix it:

I just stopped buying processed bread. Stopped. It was no longer an available option. You would be surprised at how quickly they forgot about it.

We used our toaster more. Toasted bread – any bread – was wolfed down. The children got used to the taste of the new bread. From there it was easy. It took a couple of weeks for our taste buds to adjust to the new, chewier & denser wholegrain bread. Now, it just tastes so much better. We can't go back.

Yes, you can make your own bread. This of course, is the ideal in a perfect world. I just don't. I've tried to make my own, and frankly, other people do it better than me.

Clean Foods are becoming more widely available. Not so long ago, you would have to head to your local health food shop 50 miles away to buy a good quality loaf of bread, but now most of the larger supermarkets stock a wide variety of healthy bread options. Take a bit of time to browse through the ingredient lists and find a clean bread option that suits your family.

What to look for in your bread: Your goal is find bread made with clean, natural ingredients including 100% Whole Wheat or 100% whole grain flour. No additives. The first ingredient listed in the ingredient label will be whole-wheat flour or 100% whole-wheat flour. We go through approximately five loaves of bread a week. I freeze 3 and pop two in my fridge. When needed, I pop the frozen bread in the fridge to thaw overnight.

TIP #5
Makeover your 'Usual' dinners

Dinner is the best place to start when you start eating clean. When you are making the change from a processed food lifestyle to your new, clean, real food lifestyle – don't complicate it. Start basic. You can always tweak it to suit at a later stage. Make a list of all the dinners you 'usually' make and start making Cleaner versions by replacing all elements that don't fit with your new lifestyle.

When I started I aimed to make a clean version of everything we already ate. One dish at a time, I substituted processed ingredients for a fresh, clean alternative. For example: If you have a weekly fish and chips night, make a Clean Version with fresh fish and oven baked potato chips, a squeeze of lemon and a Clean tartar sauce and don't forget to add the salad.

TIP # 6
Add ONE new recipe or dish to YOUR Menu Plan for the week (or Month. Remember, you run a home, not a Restaurant)

Starting your family on a clean eating plan is a bit like when you moved out of home and into your own place, I bet you could make, maybe 3-5 meals by heart. Build on what you know and then, once you have cleaned up your existing menu, begin introducing at least one new recipe or dish, either every week – or month – whatever suits. There are so many talented mothers who work hard to create recipes that they kindly share. Take a look at my resource page for a few of my favorite websites to find clean eating recipes.

TIP # 7
Be Prepared and Cook in bulk

Certain meals are easy to double up and freeze. Soup, Casseroles & Bolognaise sauce should NEVER be cooked in single batches – Double up when you cook and then freeze the additional serving. This gives you a 'go to meal' that you can get on the table in no time. It will save you time and sanity.

Here are some of the meals that I normally double up on when cooking. There is something warm and fuzzy fantastic about opening your freezer to find a home cooked, readymade meal that you can heat up and serve - guilt free.

Granola Cereal	*Beef Stroganoff*
Wholemeal pancakes	*Chicken Casserole*
Salmon Patties	*Chicken Pie*
Spinach and Feta Muffins	*Meatballs and tomato sauce*
Macaroni and Cheese	*Bolognaise Sauce*
Lasagne	

TIP # 8
Eat Happy Meat & DAIRY

"Happy Meat" is our family's name for meat that is organic, free range, grass-fed or wild caught. Basically, the animal had a good life before it landed on our plate. As Dr. Oz says; *"When it comes to buying [meat and] dairy products you cannot just peel or wash them like you would your produce"...so it's best to go organic.*

A few years ago, I was discussing the source of our red meat with a self sufficient farming friend of mine. All of the meat her family ate was lovingly raised on her farm and then killed (as humanely as possible). Initially I was kind of horrified. I asked her how she could bear to eat these animals, that were, in effect, her pets? Some even had names. She asked me how I could even consider eating any animal without being aware of the life it had led before it ended up on our table. I guess that stuck with me.

Choose to be accountable for the food you put on your plate. The meat our family eats is raised free range and fed food nature intended it to eat. This is not negotiable for me. If I can't find 'happy' meat and dairy, we won't eat meat until I do. Take the time to do a bit of research as to where you can get the best quality meat and dairy for your family.

Shop with Conscience. Shopping for meat in a supermarket is almost, well ... clinical. Standing in the Meat Aisle freaks me out. Neatly dressed people buying neatly wrapped portions of selective cuts. It hides the fact that an animal had to die for that beef fillet to get on our plate.

Society and our kids are missing the link between the living farm animal to what's on our dinner plate every night. I believe it's important for them to understand this connection. For some reason, pre-clean eating, I thought that this was too 'messy a talk' to have with my children. I never discussed where meat comes from.

Since changing our eating habits, it's become important for me to explain to my children how we select our meat, where it comes from and the life it had before landing on our plate.

It's had a dramatic effect on their eating choices. I have seen my kids appreciate their food more. They don't waste and they are all more open to other food group options, namely grains, fruit and vegetables. All of my children now ask what they are eating when I put food in front of them. This is a big win for me.

Diet fads come and go. High Protein. Low fat. Let's be honest, they change all the time. We don't follow any particular 'diet'. We eat from a wide range of food groups. Some of my family members choose to avoid meat and I respect that. The rest eat meat that is grass fed, free range and organically raised.

Mass-produced, factory-farmed, commercially grown meat and animal by products, whether its lamb, beef, pork, chicken or dairy products are known to be LOADED with antibiotics and hormones that are designed to cope with intensive farming conditions needed to generate the maximum amount of meat per animal (maximum amount of profit for producers too).

Be selective with the meat and dairy products you buy. Let your children know what they are eating and raise your children to be empathetic to the world around them. It all starts with you.

9 Reasons to eat LESS Meat

I know that the high protein diets are very popular at the moment, but personally, I just don't like the idea of consuming animal products in massive quantities. We eat meat around three times a week. I'm not too sure where that fits in terms of a lot or a little, but we used to eat meat daily, so I am happy with the direction we are heading as a family. It took us a while to get our heads accustomed to the idea that a meal is still a meal, even when it doesn't contain meat.

Our family supports the Meatless Monday Initiative, not only for the health benefits, but also to help do our bit for the environment. *The following information was taken directly from the Meatless Monday website. Please take a look at their website and join us in supporting it.*

Do what works for your family, but here are a few reasons why I choose to reduce the amount of meat I feed my family.

1. LOWER CANCER RISK: Hundreds of studies suggest that diets high in fruits and vegetables may reduce cancer risk. Both red and processed meat consumption are associated with colon cancer.

2. REDUCE HEART DISEASE: Recent data from a Harvard University study found that replacing saturated fat-rich foods (for example, meat and full fat dairy) with foods that are rich in polyunsaturated fat (for example, vegetable oils, nuts and seeds) reduces the risk of heart disease by 19%

3. FIGHT DIABETES: Research suggests that higher consumption of red and processed meat increase the risk of type 2 diabetes.

4. CURB OBESITY: People on low-meat or vegetarian diets have significantly lower body weights and body mass indices. A recent study from Imperial College London also found that reducing overall meat consumption can prevent long-term weight gain.

5. LIVE LONGER: Red and processed meat consumption is associated with increases in total mortality, cancer mortality and cardiovascular disease mortality.

6. IMPROVE YOUR DIET. Consuming beans or peas results in higher intakes of fibre, protein, folate, zinc, iron and magnesium with lower intakes of saturated fat and total fat.

7. REDUCE YOUR CARBON FOOTPRINT. The United Nations' Food and Agriculture Organization estimates the meat industry generates nearly one-fifth of the man-made greenhouse gas emissions that are accelerating climate change worldwide . . . far more than transportation. And annual worldwide demand for meat continues to grow. Reining in meat consumption once a week can help slow this trend.

8. MINIMIZE WATER USAGE. The water needs of livestock are tremendous, far above those of vegetables or grains. An estimated 1,800 to 2,500 gallons of water go into a single pound of beef. Soy tofu produced in California requires 220 gallons of water per pound.

9. HELP REDUCE FOSSIL FUEL DEPENDENCE. On average, about 40 calories of fossil fuel energy go into every calorie of feed lot beef in the U.S. Compare this to the 2.2 calories of fossil fuel energy needed to produce one calorie of plant-based protein. Moderating meat consumption is a great way to cut fossil fuel demand.

SOURCE http://www.meatlessmonday.com/about-us/why-meatless/

TIP #9
Save money and Sanity by Eating Vegetables and Fruit that are in season.

Ideally the vegetables and fruit you eat should be local and if possible, organic (this should not be a deal breaker. Budget often does determine the quality we can afford to get). Please don't be hard on yourself. There are many times when 'organic' is not in my price range, but I do endeavour to buy local as much as I can.

Farmers markets and most supermarkets now stock a local range. Support your local economy by buying local. Shop with the season, which typically means what is on sale. This is also a good way to ensure that your family gets to try a greater range of fruits and vegetables – naturally.

Buy in bulk, prepare and freeze. If green beans are on special – buy for the month. Divide into serving sizes and freeze – ready for the next meal.

TIP #10
Drink More Water.

65% of your body is just plain old water. We need water. Every single day.

Getting my children to drink more water was easy. I just stopped buying soda and cordial. It was just not an option in our home. When your child is thirsty; offer them water. Start early by putting water in their sippy cups or bottle. Ditch the juice today.

The Benefits of Drinking more Water.

- Keep metabolism regular
- Decrease food cravings
- Help burn fat in your body
- Important in maintaining muscle tone
- Increased energy levels
- Clear skin as water helps the body flush toxins from the body and improves the flow of blood to the skin.
- Increases the production of new blood and muscle cells
- Firmer skin as cells are not dehydrated.
- Regular Bowel movements
- Eliminates toxins in your body
- Your lungs are moistened by water. Water helps you breathe. When you don't drink enough water, your histamine levels increase. This can lead to allergies and asthma.

- It's better for your teeth and that means fewer fillings and fewer dentist bills.
- PLUS $$ Save money by not having to buy soda and other sugary drinks.

Every single cell in your body requires water to function effectively. Without water, we start to waste away.

Maybe I take this to extremes, but this is how I structured getting our water drinking habit in place:

1. We drink a glass of water in the morning when we wake up (1 cup)
2. Every day, I give each of my children a 600ml water bottle which they generally finish by the time they get home from school or kindy (equivalent to about 3 cups of water).
3. I serve water with a snack when they get home from school (1cup)
4. And we all drink water with dinner (1 more cup)
5. In addition to this, on hot days and after school sports days, they will still drink when they are thirsty. This is just my way of ensuring that they get into the habit of drinking water regularly. Your body quickly adjusts to this routine and you actually start recognizing thirst and craving water.

If your child has a problem skin with breakouts and redness, you will be amazed at the difference this little change will make.

A Super cool idea to try: One of the best things about water is that you can see right through it. Try adding some pieces of fruit to your ice block trays. Pop the fruity ice blocks in water and instantly transform your standard water into something a little bit fancy.

"Before I got married I had six theories about raising children; now, I have six children and no theories."

— John Wilmot

THE 6 BIGGEST PROBLEMS WE ENCOUNTERED WHEN WE STARTED CLEAN EATING WITH KIDS

Problem #1.
Eating More.

Kids are always hungry. Always. I can feed them the biggest breakfast and yet on our way out the door, at least one will tell me they are still hungry. Without fail.

Keeping clean, healthy snacks on hand means you won't resort to the fastest (often unhealthiest) options. I had to work snacks into our diet very early on in the clean eating process. I went from three meals a day to six planned meals a day. Don't get me wrong, we always did snack in the day, but I never really counted it. I never planned for it and I almost always resorted to a bag of biscuits, chips or other junk food in a bag.

To help me out with this, I now keep a Snack Box in my pantry and snack box in my fridge. Once a week I will fill it with homemade granola bars, little bags of popcorn; peanut biscuits, nuts and seeds etc. It's the same box that I resort to for school lunch box snacks. In the fridge, I keep fruit, sliced carrots, celery and muffins. Make it easy to grab healthy food.

The more you can get your children to full up on healthy, whole foods the less inclined they will be to grab for the unhealthy stuff.

Problem #2.
What should we eat now?

Overnight, I had nothing to cook. All my 'regular' meals were tainted with processed elements. I used instant gravy, canned soup mixes, pre-made meals, bottled sauces. Now what?

I started small by remaking our usual meals using only fresh, whole foods. I pretty much had to learn how to cook. No more packet gravies or instant meals for me.

After a while, my family started getting bored of me rotating the five dishes I knew how to cook, so I began introducing one new meal a week and began keeping a recipe book full of meals and snacks. I'm not exactly fond of cooking, so my focus is still on fast food – but now it's healthy too.

Problem #3.
Changing how I shopped.

They should teach a class at school called 'Economics of shopping 101'. It's one of the biggest household expenses and accounts for a massive dent in our household income and yet I have operated it like an amateur for the past 20 years.

Shopping involves comparing prices, budgeting, meal preparation and often quite a bit of time and research (aka browsing through those supermarket mailers that arrive like magic your mail box the day before your weekly shopping trip).

Over the years, to make the process easier, I have followed a well oiled shopping routine: grab the largest trolley or shopping basket and head down the neatly arranged aisle – following the profitable path laid out for me by the Supermarket Super Marketers, all the while buying my 'regular' brands (or the one I saw on TV) and, of course, never ever missing an aisle.

When you change your eating habits, you need to rethink how you shop.

6 Supermarket Shopping Tricks I learned the hard way.

1. Make a list of everything you need for the week and stick to it. It is so very easy to fall for the promotional up sells offered around every corner. You decide what goes into your trolley because ultimately that is what ends up in your pantry and on your family's plate.

2. Avoid (or rush through at hyper speed) the center aisles of the grocery store. The fresh, clean foods are normally located along the edges where the refrigerators are located. Remember, the good stuff has a use by date.

3. Don't shop when you are hungry. EVER! It is hard to make good purchasing decisions when you are hungry. The human body is designed to refuel fast when hungry. Your brain will make any full fat, sugar laded carbohydrate look delicious. A hungry body and brain is not your friend in the Supermarket.

4. Take cash with you so you can't splurge on your budget. This one sends me into a bit of a sweat but it is the best way I have of controlling my spending. If I have cash in my pocket, then I am limited in how much I spend. I get very embarrassed when I don't have enough money at the checkout so I use this in my favour to force me to buy what's on my shopping list.

5. Learn to read the label. If you don't recognize or know what's in it - leave it on the shelf. If your ancestors wouldn't recognize it as food – then chances are it not good enough to serve to your family. Set your standards high regarding the food you feed them.

6. Shop once a week only. This saves you money and time. The reason I shop once a week is that it is pretty much the limit on how long my vegetables and fruit stay fresh. A weekly shopping trip and a weekly meal plan are doable for me. I can plan 7 days' worth of meals and my fridge and freezer can hold about a weeks' worth of food. This timeline works for me, but I encourage you to decide on a system that fits with your family.

Problem #4.
Getting Organized

Changing to a Clean Eating lifestyle meant I had to get organized. We had to restructure our pantry and fridge and throw out all processed, crappy foods we had in our kitchen.

Meal planning and food preparation became part of my weekly chores. In the beginning it was hard, but now it definitely makes life easier. I can shop more effectively and there is no more of the 5pm 'What shall I make for dinner' panic. Breakfasts and school lunches are now so easy to put together; even the kids can prepare them before school.

Problem #5.
No More Takeout

It's Day 1. of your new clean eating lifestyle. It's 5.00pm (For most parents, this is one hellish time of day). You haven't been back at home since you left it at 8.00am that morning.

Kids have been at school and afternoon sports. Everyone is tired and hungry. It would be so, so, so easy to swing past [Fill in the space] fast food outlet. How do you NOT succumbing to take out foods?

The first week was hard. I wasn't prepared for the last minute rush and I resorted to quite a few egg meals. I can pretty much cook any egg perfectly now. Whew!

How to avoid the 5.00pm take out dash when you are tired and kids are whining, grumpy and hungry.

5 Five o'clock Coping Strategies

1. Keep a well stocked kitchen. This is a bit easier said than done. A well stocked kitchen simply means that you always have something available to eat. It requires planning and organization. I am not naturally blessed with either of those skills. I need to work a bit harder at keeping my pantry organized. When I do get this right, it does make it easy to eat clean.

2. Always have a couple of pre-made meals in the freezer. Spaghetti Sauce is my No 1 go-to meal of all time. Reheat and serve with some fresh pasta and you have a meal in minutes.

3. Double up on recipes and freeze. If you take nothing out of this book except this little tip, it would have been worth its purchase price: ALWAYS make and freeze extra serves so that you have your own readymade meals for when you need them. Most one pot meals like casseroles, soups & pasta sauces can be doubled with minimum fuss. I use disposable 1 liter freezer containers and try double up on at least two meals a week.

4. Learn some quick, easy meals that you know you can pull together in a matter of minutes. Most of the recipes I have included in this book will fit into that category. I am not a massive fan of cooking, so I try keeping it simple where I can.

5. If you know you are going to be late home – invest in a slow cooker /Crockpot and have a hot, ready to eat meal available for when you get home. I had my slow cooker gathering dust in my cupboard for about two years before I used it. Now it would be one of the things I grabbed on my way out the door if we had a house fire.

Problem #6.Our Biggest Problem (by Far)
My children didn't like vegetables.

My Kids were NOT used to eating fresh, whole foods and they let me know it!

Their palates had been trained (I have to take the blame for this) to like commercially produced, chemical enhanced flavors - with added sugar. I had created a problem and I had to fix it. Teaching my children to eat vegetables was, I hate to admit it, damn hard.

Prior to clean eating, I only served my children the foods I knew they would eat. It was easier. No tantrums, no crying and dinner got eaten. But, I also knew, that at some point, I would have to face the predicament I was creating. Chicken nuggets and apple slices do not look so cute on your teenager's plate.

Whenever we went to the grandparent's house or friends for dinner, I would feel stressed. I didn't want my kids to 'expose me' and let on that they didn't eat their vegetables. No mother likes to admit this.

When we started eating clean, I was lucky as two of my four children ate almost everything. They naturally liked vegetables and fruit. I had it easy with them. Ironically, I didn't even know that they weren't fussy eaters. I never gave them a chance.

The other two, however, made dinner time a nightmare. We had days of tantrums, gagging and tears – all over a little bit of broccoli. It did get better. It took about three weeks to go from gagging over broccoli to eating it without even a grimace. ALL my kids now eat their vegetables. They don't have to like it; they just have to eat it.

Let me just say, on a primal, selfish level - I LOVE the feeling I get from watching all of my children munch through a pile of veggies without hesitation. No fuss, no arguments. In the event you have let things slide as much as I had, the next chapter will give you some tips on how to get your children to eat their vegetables. Try one, try them all, but most of all - don't quit!

MURPHY'S LAW TO CLEAN EATING CLEARLY AND IRREVOCABLY STATES:

"REAL LIFE HAPPENS".

There will be THOSE DAYS - with movie nights and chocolate, birthday cakes and Halloween, the odd bakery dash, a decadent pudding or a night out with friends. Don't be hard on your family or yourself. Your goal is to get your family eating whole, real foods as part of their lifestyle – Even if it's only MOST OF THE TIME!!!

In our family, one of our weaknesses is tomato ketchup and chocolate – standing out like a sore thumb in my refrigerator. It's organic, but not 100% clean, but damn, childhood wouldn't be the same without it. If you can find a clean replacement for milk chocolate – please send me the recipe ASAP!

Find your happy place. Do what works for you and your family

"Sometimes the questions are complicated and the answers are simple."

Dr. Seuss

HOW TO GET YOUR KIDS TO EAT THEIR VEGETABLES

This is the #1 most frequently asked question that I get from Parents – *How can I get my child to eat their vegetables?*

There are so many opinions on this, ranging from "Let them do it in their own time" to "Make them eat it or else!". I am sure most parents have tried a bit of both. I know I have. I also enjoy the benefit of having four kids to test out my theories. So here is my two cents opinion on the subject.

Two of my children will pretty much eat any fruits and veggies I put on their plate – including brussle sprouts (these bring my husband and other two kids to breaking point). Just as with adults, some kids have a natural aversion to certain foods. There are a couple of things that don't go down well, for example: My eldest daughter eats everything – except potato. I know. Potato! We have tried to prepare it in many ways – It's not the taste that is an issue, she simply doesn't like the texture of the soft potato on her tongue.

Our solution was to make crispy oven baked potato 'chips'. I think that as she gets older, the texture issue will change – but until then, I'm willing to let this one go as I know she generally loves to eat everything.

Now my two fussy eaters are a whole other story. They have mentally prepared themselves to dislike any new food that comes from the fruit and veggie food group.

There are CHOOSING not to eat the food on their plate. In both of their cases, I am not as forgiving. I play hardball. I think we eat common vegetables. These are foods most people have access to, they are generally locally grown and in season most of the year. I do expect my children to learn to eat the veggies that are commonplace in our home.

A few vegetables that I serve most often in our home are:

Green Beans	*Pumpkin*	*Cauliflower*
Peas	*Potato*	*Broccoli*
Spinach	*Sweet potato*	*Corn*
Cabbage	*Zucchini*	*Celery*
Carrots		

There are others, but these are the featured regulars. I am more forgiving when my children decide that they don't like an exotic vegetable, artichoke or eggplant come to mind, but I do think that my children should eat from the list above without a fuss and give everything else a good go.

13 TIPS ON HOW TO GET YOUR KIDS TO EAT REAL FOOD (WITHOUT A FUSS)

Some kids take to vegetables like a duck to water, while others come to the table kicking and screaming. If your children are of the *kicking and screaming* variety (I have two of them), then here are my tips on getting them to eat real food.

Feed your babies real food as soon as they begin eating solids.

Avoid store bought baby food. I believe this was my first mistake. My first and fourth children (the two non fussy eaters) were fed homemade food. With my first, I had the time and with the fourth, I was just lazy, so he got to eat what everyone else ate. My middle two children were not so fortunate; I bought 'organic' store stocked baby food to save time. Don't be fooled by the marketing hype - It's NOT the same as the real thing. It did not prepare their taste buds for real food and I believe that it was the start to their fussy eating issues.

Don't 'Give up' if your child rejects a food you serve.

Fussy eating is common in childhood. Many kids don't like change. Often, a child needs to be exposed to a new food up to 3-5 times before they will accept it into their diet.

As parents we tend to surrender when a child decides they don't like a type of food. More often than we would like to admit, we create the monster by offering them something else to replace the uneaten food, or we never serve that food again once it has been rejected. Keep going. Just keep putting it on their plate and insist that they try 'just two bites'.

My son had an issue with broccoli. An apocalyptic issue with it. He would gag, cry, throw a massive 'tanty' and generally make dinner time a nightmare.

At first, I tried to force him to eat by threatening him with taking away all sorts of his favorite things. It was stressing the entire family out. So, I changed my tactic. I still put it on his plate, but I just asked him to take two bites. I didn't judge over the size of the bites (trust me, in the beginning they were mice size bites). I rewarded any effort with "Well done". Broccoli became a regular vegetable at dinner and his bites gradually got bigger. I began to focus on how little was left on his plate "Oh my gosh, you almost ate half". It took us less than one week to go from gagging to finishing the broccoli on his plate. My son now eats broccoli, celery, spinach, cabbage, corn etc.

On a side note, siblings are naturally competitive. If you praise one, the others work damn hard to get your attention on their plate. My other fussy child was so focused on 'beating' her brother that she ate her veggies purely to make her brother look bad. Hmmm. Might have to watch that one.

Texture matters.
A crispy green, raw bean vs. a mashed, soggy bean is not the same. Taste is different, texture is different even though it is the same vegetable. When introducing a new vegetable or fruit – try serving it in different ways. Once your child is familiar with it, they will accept it as part of their diet – then you can experiment with preparation. It loses its power and becomes just another thing on their plate.

No More Choices.
Everyone in our family now eats the same meal. Cook once for everyone. If they don't eat it they go hungry. Trust me; kids don't like to go hungry. They catch on really quickly that there are no options and they will eat.   Its not optional and there are no alternatives. Eat or go hungry. Period.

Limit Snack Portions.
Earlier in the book I spoke about adding planned snacks to your children's diet. Let me be clear – SNACKS are SNACKS! Don't let your child full up on too much food before dinner. They need to get to that dinner table ready to eat. They should be hungry in time for dinner, breakfast or lunch. If your kids aren't hungry, then perhaps change the portion size you are feeding them at snack times.

Prepare your Food with love.
Your children need to know that you took time and effort to create the meal you are serving them. Let them know that it makes you happy when they eat the food you made. Dinnertime is where you teach your children good eating habits, table manners and gratitude.

Turn the TV off.
Children are excellent mimics. They learn from example. If you want your children to eat their vegetables, practice good manners and develop good eating habits, then let them see you do it too. Turn off the TV, sit down and share a meal with your children.

SIMPLY Offer your Kids more real Food
It's up to you to offer your children the right choices. Obviously, if you ask them to choose between an apple or chocolate bar, odds are that chocolate bar is going down! Don't offer the chocolate bar. Present them with fresh, real food and you may be delightfully surprised at their response.

Serve it with a Dip.
I'm not kidding. Hummus, apple sauce, peanut butter or sour cream. We are talking magic, folks. It's amazing what kids will eat if they can dip it in something. Don't be scared to try out new things like celery and apple sauce and carrots and peanut butter.

Candles.
Candlelight makes everything look more appealing - even dinner and bad dates (ha ha). If I'm about to dish up a new dish, and I know that kids will put up a fight over the 'green' content, I turn off the lights and we eat by candle light. Try it!!!

Let them help with Food Preparation.
Chopping beans, dishing up, stirring a pot, setting the table and washing up. It's all part of being a family and sharing the experience of meal preparation. You are teaching your children lifetime skills that they will take to their own dinner tables one day.

Make it Fun.
Kids learn through play. The more fun you can make it – the better. We stepped this up for my daughter's 12th birthday party. We decided on a Fear Factor™ party theme. Kids delighted in trying every vegetable concoction we put in front of them – it was an awesome party where everyone tried to outdo the other – we're talking steamed spinach and anchovies (aka raw fish on rotton seaweed), boiled prunes (aka pickled cockroach), cold pumpkin (this one was the worst!).

Set a Good Example.
Let your children see you eating well. Children learn by watching what we do. Sit down with your children and eat together. Let them see you eating clean, healthy food.

The important this to remember is that it is possible to get your child to eat vegetables. You are not alone. Most parents have an issue with this to some degree – despite what they may admit to.

"If you don't take care of your body, where are you going to live?"

~Unknown

ARE ORGANIC FOODS REALLY BETTER FOR YOU?

The simple answer is YES, although the 'professionals' research results are mixed as to the degree of benefit. Generally, most agree that non organic produce contain a lower nutrient content and more pesticide residue, but that it should not stop you from eating non organic produce. The argument as to whether non organic goods are actually bad for you is still up for debate.

A survey done by the Environmental Working Group (EWG) found that many children consume up to 10 times more than the Environmental Protection Agencies (EPA) 'safe dose' of pesticides and herbicides.

The EWG put together a list of fruit and vegetables that they call the Dirty Dozen. According to them, by buying organic versions of these, you could reduce your family's exposure to pesticides and herbicides by as much as 80%. They followed this up with a Clean Fifteen list of produce which when tested, contained relatively low pesticide residue, so purchasing the non organic versions of these would be considered safe.

We try to eat organic where possible, but often budget is an issue, so we follow their Dirty Dozen and Clean Fifteen guidelines. The following was taken from the Environmental Working Group website (www.ewg.org).

EWG's Dirty Dozen™ list of produce:

1. *apples,*
2. *strawberries,*
3. *grapes,*
4. *celery,*
5. *peaches,*
6. *spinach,*
7. *sweet bell peppers,*
8. *imported nectarines,*
9. *cucumbers,*
10. *cherry tomatoes,*
11. *imported snap peas and*
12. *potatoes.*

When tested, each of these foods contained a number of different pesticide residues and showed high concentrations of pesticides relative to other produce items. Here is a quick summary of results:

Every sample of imported nectarines and 99 percent of apple samples tested positive for at least one pesticide residue. The average potato had more pesticides by weight than any other food.

A single grape sample contained 15 pesticides. Single samples of celery, cherry tomatoes, imported snap peas and strawberries showed 13 different pesticides apiece.

The Clean Fifteen™

These fifteen fruits and vegetables are known as the Clean Fifteen. Relatively few pesticides were detected on these foods, and tests found low total concentrations of pesticides. EWG's Clean Fifteen™ for 2014 - the produce least likely to hold pesticide residues - are:

1. *avocados,*
2. *sweet corn,*
3. *Pineapples,*
4. *cabbage,*
5. *frozen sweet peas,*
6. *onions,*
7. *Asparagus,*
8. *mangoes,*
9. *papayas,*
10. *Kiwis,*
11. *eggplant,*
12. *grapefruit,*
13. *cantaloupe,*
14. *cauliflower and*
15. *sweet potatoes.*

"The most important thing is to enjoy your life—to be happy—it's all that matters."

— Audrey Hepburn

LET"S TALK ABOUT SUGAR

Is Sugar really that bad for you?

Is the massive hype about Sugar really necessary? Is it really the big bad wolf that the experts are making it out to be? Our body needs sugar, but not all sugar is created equal. The problem is that too many of us are eating the wrong kind of sugar and way too much of it.

The Science behind Sugar in our Body (the very basics)

The body needs energy to function. We get most of that energy from carbohydrates in our food. Carbohydrates are broken down into simple sugars, which are absorbed into the bloodstream. As the sugar level rises in our blood, the pancreas releases the hormone insulin, which is needed to move sugar from the blood into the cells, where the sugar can be used as energy.

For kids over 2 years old, 50% to 60% of calories should be coming from carbohydrates. The key is to make sure that they come from good sources of carbohydrates and that they are not getting too much for their bodies to handle effectively.

There are two major forms of carbohydrates:

1. Simple carbohydrates (or simple sugars): these include fructose, glucose, and lactose, which also are found in nutritious whole fruits and honey (we will touch on this one below) and
2. Complex carbohydrates (or starches): found in foods such as vegetables, grains, rice, and breads and cereals

The health problems we are seeing now is that too much of our carbohydrate intake is in the form of simple sugars. Our bodies were not designed to consume a large supply of simple sugars. We are meant to get the majority of our energy from complex carbohydrates which are broken down within our body at a slower rate, releasing energy at a steady pace. This allows our cells to use and distribute the sugar produced more effectively, without over stressing them.

10 Reasons to Avoid too much Sugar

1. Weakens the immune system: Consuming 100g sugar a day (2 ½ cans of soda) reduces the ability of the white blood cells in our blood to kill germs and bacteria by 40% - 50%.
2. Increases acidity in the body
3. Decreases tissue elasticity and function (an increase in cellulite in girls).
4. Cause of diabetes.
5. Linked to ADHD in children.
6. Increases tooth decay.
7. Increase risk of obesity: An extra sugary drink each day increase a child's risk of obesity by 60% (source: The Lancet 2001)
8. Children are more sensitive to the effects of sugar than adults. A study comparing the sugar response in children and adults showed that adrenaline levels in children remained ten times higher than normal for up to five hours after a test dose of sugar.

The effects are even more pronounced in younger children which may be related to their brains growing more rapidly in preschool years.

9. Decreases learning performance.
10. Hyperactivity.

How to Reduce the Sugar in your children's Diet

Be Aware of the hidden sugar.

It is important that you monitor the amount of sugar your children are eating, however, it's not always as obvious as a spoon of the stuff sprinkled on their porridge. Most processed foods contain refined sugar. I'm not just talking about candy either. Packaged foods such as flavored yogurt, children's cereal, pizza, ketchup and bread are often hiding added sugar. Read the ingredients before you add it to your children's plates.

Substitute with the good stuff.

Replace all refined white sugar with raw sugar, or even better: honey, apple sauceor pure maple syrup. My theory is this: Sweetened foods are generally a treat. They are not to be consumed in massive quantities. If you are going to use sugar or sweetener in your cooking or baking, at least make sure that it contains some nutrient value.

Start Right.

Commercial breakfast cereals and fruit juices are two of the biggest culprits when it comes to finding hidden sugar in your children's diet.

Immediately cut their daily sugar intake by starting each morning with a sugar free breakfast. Aim for a high protein, complex carbohydrate breakfast to get your child's system firing on full. Start your child's day off strong and serve up an egg on wholemeal toast or a bowl of homemade Muesli and yogurt.

What about the sugar in fruit and Natural Sweeteners?

The sugar found in whole fruits (called fructose) is a simple sugar which our body can process quickly. It means that the sugar in fruit is made available as energy in our cells really quickly; however, fruits are also high in nutrients, minerals and fiber which are also needed by our bodies to operate effectively.

There is a bit of a debate around this issue, but personally, I am not going to stop giving my children apples to eat because of their sugar content. Unlike Commercial Food Manufacturers, I am inclined to trust that Mother Nature has packed the perfect amount of sugar in each fruit. I believe that the benefits of eating a nutrient packed, fiber, full whole fruit far outweigh the issue of it containing sugar.

Similarly with honey and natural sweeteners, at the end of the day, they are still a sugar. I do use these in my cooking, but I am in control the amount that goes into our food, so I am able to limit the amount that my children eat in the day.

Life expectancy would grow by leaps and bounds if green vegetables smelled as good as bacon."

~Doug Larson

EATING CLEAN ON A BUDGET (EVEN A VERY SMALL BUDGET)

Our family operates off one income. Our budget is tight and, like most families, our life is busy – but Clean Eating is still doable. Cost is one of the major reasons that many families don't eat Clean. Fast Foods are often readily available and cheap so they fit into budget and time constraints a little bit too easily.

Here are 12 ways we work clean eating into our Budget:

1. I make meals and snacks (biscuits, muffins and granola bars) from scratch. By not buying pre-made meals and packaged treats, you actually save. Yes, I know it takes a bit of time in the kitchen, but you are there anyway, you might as well pop a tray of muffins in the oven whilst you are cooking dinner.

2. We use cheaper cuts of meat – whole chicken, chicken thighs, gravy beef etc – these make for a tastier casserole anyway.

3. Buy vegetables and fruit that are in season. Seasonal food is cheaper. Get creative with what's available.

4. Shop at your local farmers markets. Not only is it cheaper and fresher, but you are supporting your local community too.

5. I cook in bulk – double up on some meals so that you don't have to cook twice.

6. Bulk up most dishes with vegetables. Pumpkin, potatoes, sweet potatoes and tomatoes are perfect for this.

7. Snack on Popcorn. It is easy to make, cheap, whole grain and kids love it.

8. Get familiar with your shopping list and the contents of your pantry. Buy in bulk when items are on special and don't buy what you won't actually use.

9. Use canned goods where you can. Organic tomatoes and apple puree are always in my pantry. It saves me buying tomatoes and apples when they go up to $7/kg. Agh!

10. Can't afford to buy organic? Use the Dirty Dozen list as a guide and go organic with these. Remember, you could be cutting your exposure to harmful pesticides by up to 80% just by doing this. Most of the vegetables on the Dirty Dozen list are actually easy to grow. A small vegetable garden can yield you an organic salad for around 25c per salad. You can't get much cheaper than that!

11. Invest in a couple of Chickens. OK, so maybe I don't save much money by having a couple of backyard hens. I figure we come out about even, but it is so worth the effort. Our two feathered girls – Ms Flo and Ms Pepper

provide us with an endless amount of joy and an average of 10 eggs a week. It's an experience that your children will cherish forever.

12. Drink water. Immediately cut out spending on juices, soda, cordial etc.

Five of our Favorite Frugal Family Dinners

No matter how careful we try to be, there are often more than a few days in the month when we have more month left over than money. The easiest way to stretch out our income is by saving on our food bill.

Here are Five Frugal Meals that I cook when times are a bit lean. I keep all ingredients for these five meals in my pantry or freezer, so I know that I always have a meal on hand when times get a bit lean.

1. Spaghetti Bolognaise
2. Lasagna
3. Roast Chicken, Rice and Vegetables & Gravy
4. Chinese Rice
5. Beef & Vegetable Casserole

You can find all of these recipes in Part 2 of this book.

How we eat Happy Meat on a Budget

I mentioned earlier that eating Happy Meat was not negotiable for us. Animal welfare is one of our biggest family priorities. By choosing to eat organic, free range meat, I have to make the following compromises to fit it into our budget:

1. I buy the cheaper cuts: Budget meat cuts are minced meat, whole chickens, stewing beef and chicken drumsticks.
2. We don't eat meat every night (around 3 times a week including chicken). If you feed your family meat every night, then I would recommend getting into the habit of implementing a 'meatless' dinner at least once a week.
3. I bulk up most meals with vegetables.
4. I buy in bulk when possible then repackage into serving sizes and freeze.

"Trust yourself. You know more than you think you do."

— Benjamin Spock

WHAT SHOULD WE BE FEEDING OUR CHILDREN?

Keep it Simple: A little Bit of Everything

We could discuss the hundreds of different food theories, or we could just keep it simple. When I feed my kids I try to include a portion of each food group at every meal. Maybe it's a bit oversimplified, but I work on making sure that around half the meal consists of fruit and vegetables. This little plate graphic below is pretty much what I try and stick to, but I don't over think it too much.

There is a lot (and I do mean a lot!) of variation in what the professionals say regarding how much we should be feeding our children. It can drive you a bit crazy if you go too deep into it.

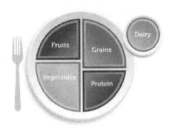

Daily Food Group portions by age

Kids do vary in size and appetite, so this table is a recommendation only. Every child is different, so do what works for your child regarding portion sizes, but aim to include a bit from each food group. After a day spent reading every nutritionist blog I could find, this is what I came up the – the general consensus regarding number of servings you should be feeding your child. To be fair, I have one child who eats more along the minimum recommended servings and another who is skirting on the maximum.

Ages (in years)	1-3	4-7	8-11	10-12	Suggestions
Grains, Bread & Cereals	2-3	3-5	4-6	5-7	Granola, Wholemeal pasta, wholemeal bread, rice
Fruits	1	2	2-3	2-3	Whole fruit, canned fruit in natural juices, fresh juice
Vegetables	1½– 2	2-4	3-5	4-9	Whole vegetables, raw or cooked, salad, legumes. NOTE: I do include potatoes in here, but this is restricted to 1 serve.
Dairy (Cheese Yogurt & Dairy Alternatives)	3	2-3	2-3	3-5	Milk, yogurt, cheese, cream cheese, cottage cheese
Lean Meat / Protein	½ - 1	½ - 1	1-1½	1-2	Cooked meat, chicken or fish (canned included), tofu, legumes such as lentils, chick peas, eggs
Fats	Fat is naturally found in a lot of the food we eat, but I still allow butter, oils, coconut oils & nuts to contribute to our diet. I try to keep these to 1-2 serves a day across all age groups				

Basic outline showing Number of Servings of each food group per day.

"If you can't pronounce it, don't eat it"

~Common sense

PORTION CONTROL: HOW MUCH SHOULD WE BE FEEDING OUR KIDS?

Portion control plays an important part in a healthy diet. Weight loss industry gurus will tell you to weigh it up or count the calories, but really, all you need is your own hand.

How to use your hand to measure your portion size:

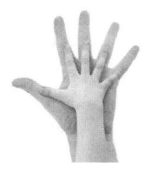

Your palm size = your protein portions such as meats or fish
Your fist size = veggie portions.
Your cupped hand size = carbohydrate portions, fruit, dairy (yogurt and milk) and also snack size portion.
Your thumb size = fat portions like butter or cheese.

The great thing about this simple hand system is that it works no matter what your child's age, because their hands grow along with their appetites. How cool is that?

Take a look at the image below showing the change in fast food portion sizes from 1955. The child size drink alone increased by close to 60% in size from 1955 to 2002.

It's not a surprise that we are overestimating how much food we should be putting on our plates.

Fast Food Portion Sizes 1955 - 2002

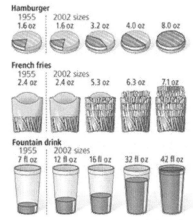

Source: Harvard Medical School Website.

Based on data from the Journal of the American Dietetic Association

"Sometimes life knocks you on your ass... get up, get up, get up!!! Happiness is not the absence of problems; it's the ability to deal with them."

— Steve Maraboli, Life, the Truth, and Being Free

REDISCOVER YOUR HUNGER CUES

Our bodies are truly amazing biological machines. We all have an inbuilt system which alerts us to when we need food and water – and when we have had enough. These are called Hunger Cues.

One of the reasons that many people struggle to maintain a healthy weight is that they have lost the ability to recognize their body's signals that tell them when they are hungry or when they are full. As you begin to eat clean you will begin to notice these signs more clearly. Your children will be hungry at the appropriate times and they will learn to distinguish between hunger and thirst cues.

Babies are a perfect example of these skills in action. They follow their hunger signals naturally. When their bodies tell them they're hungry, they cry or fuss and when they have had enough, they stop eating. By the time they reach around three years of age, distractions start to get in the way of this natural way of eating.

Over time, outside influences begin to affect us and we lose the skill of recognizing our body's hunger signals.

Food is everywhere—in grocery stores, Television commercials kitchen pantry, fridge, Mom's handbag - to name just a few. It can be hard to pay attention to your hunger signals with all of this happening around you.

Changing bad eating habits are just as important as introducing good habits when embarking on a healthy lifestyle. Teaching your children to recognize and respond appropriately to their bodies hunger cues is part of process.

Does your Family Have Any of These Bad Eating Habits?

Skipping Meals.
Don't skip meals. Skipping breakfast because you are late for school means that by the time when lunchtime hits, you're extra hungry and eat more than you should (often more of the wrong stuff too).

Distractions.
You may watch TV, read, or use the computer while you eat. As a Mom, I am often guilty of snacking while I cook. This stops you paying attention to what or how much you have eaten and may distract you to the point that you miss your body telling you that you are full enough to stop eating.

Eating too fast.
Slow down your meal so that your food has time to reach your stomach and signal your brain that you have had enough. Eating too fast will result in you consuming too much before your body has time to let you know that it is full. It takes approximately 20 minutes for fullness signals to transmit from the stomach back to the brain. So, if you eat too fast it's easy to override this system and eat more than what the body needs.

Comfort eating.

From early in life we get taught to relate food to joy and comfort. Attaching emotion to food is another reason that people fail to recognize their hunger cues. Are you or your children eating because you are bored, sad or tired or just out of habit?

Large Portions.

Research shows that when people are given larger portions, they eat more. Control the portion sizes you put on your children's plates. Teach them to recognize what an adequate portion size is for their age.

Don't worry. Your hunger and fullness signals are still there. You just have to learn how to tune into them again. Ditch the TV dinners. Turn the TV off and eat together as a family. The best way to break bad habits is to replace them with new, healthy and empowering habits.

Here are 4 Healthy Eating Habits you can put in place today.

1. Eat regularly. Don't skip meals as this leads to binging on bad food choices.

2. Be Conscious of the food you are eating. Turn off the TV and at the table to eat your meals as a family.

3. Focus on changing one thing at a time. Set yourself small achievable goals. Choose and change one thing at a time. For example: If you want your family to drink more water, the get rid of the soda and cordial in your home. Get everyone a good drink bottle and fill your fridge with bottles of cold, clean water. Make it easy to break the bad habit of drinking sugary drinks.

4. Stop using Food as a Reward. Are you rewarding your children with food. Using food dissociates food with hunger. Don't give your children food to settle or stop them crying. Like Pavlov and his dog studies, this leads to a link between emotional eating later in life. Choose non-food related rewards such as family outings, computer time, a board game with mom or dad.

"It's bizarre that the produce manager is more important to my children's health than the pediatrician."

— Meryl Streep

THE ART OF CLEAN SNACKING

The whole world is screaming at you to "stop eating so much!", and here I am telling you to feed your children more.

Think of snacks as mini meals that help provide your kids with the nutrients and energy they need to play and grow. Children have smaller stomachs and snacking allows their bodies to absorb nutrients regularly throughout the day.

A big part of Clean Eating is eating more good food, not less. This means including planned healthy snacks in your day.

Set regular snack times.
Teach your children to choose snacks that are good for them. I recommend choosing snacks rich in protein, contain a healthy fat and served with a vegetable or fruit.

Eating every few hours is beneficial for:

- stabilizing blood sugar,
- maintaining weight and actually aiding weightless,

- increasing energy throughout the day
- enhancing your mood
- allows you to control the food you put into your body
- Snacks keep you from getting hungry and overeating at mealtimes or making bad food choices.

13 Clean Eating Snacks that Kids love to Eat.

- Popcorn – We have a popcorn maker we bought off Gumtree for around $15. I use it all the time.
- Fresh Veggies & Dip – chopped veggies, ready to eat with cottage cheese, hummus, pureed apple or peanut butter.
- Peanut Butter and whole wheat crackers.
- Nuts and dried fruit
- Muffins, Muffins and More muffins. So easy and versatile. Savoury or sweet, they fit into lunch boxes and freeze beautifully. See our favourite recipes in part 2.
- Granola Bars
- Homemade biscuits
- Fruit – Nature's takeaway.
- Hard boiled eggs
- Cup of fresh seasonal fruit and yogurt
- Fruit and a handful of nuts
- Fruit juice Icy Pops

- Apple Slinkies – Apples that have been cored and made into a slinky. I got this off Ebay for $10 and it is brilliant. It turns the ordinary apple into a slinky. Overnight, Apples became a high commodity in our home. Google 'Apple Peeler Corer machine' and you will see what I mean. BEST BUY EVER!

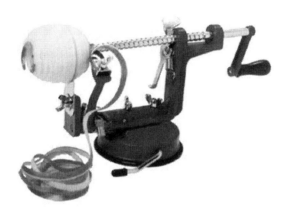

The Brilliant Apple Slinky Machine It Peels, Cores and slices an apple in seconds! I may sound like a lunchtime infomercial, but I Love it! We even take this little guy camping with us. It is so easy to whip up an apple slinky for everyone. You can set it to peel or leave the peel on. You can watch a video on how it works on my website www.cleaneatingwithkids.com/appleslinky

PUTTING IT ALL TOGETHER

Ok. You have had enough of the crap that your kids are eating and you have decided to overhaul your lifestyle. You should have a good idea of what clean eating is about and hopefully a few tips up your sleeve on how to make the process that little bit easier.

If you are the type of person who likes to skim through a book by checking out the chapter headings and summaries, then this is for you.

My Little Summary on How to Eat Clean with Kids:

1. Skip the food with Numbers in their ingredients list.
2. The fewer ingredients the better (think 3 - 5 at most).
3. Eat for health.
4. Drink Water every day.
5. Be aware of your portion sizes
6. Replace the processed food with real, whole foods
7. Choose happy meat and eat with conscience.
8. Shop local and eat seasonal.
9. Always eat breakfast.
10. Plan your meals.
11. ***And Finally …. Simply eat real food most of the time.***

PART 2

KID FRIENDLY CLEAN EATING RECIPES

14 Fast & Easy Clean Breakfast Recipes

Scrambled Eggs on Toast
Wholemeal Banana Pancakes, Vanilla Yogurt & Maple Syrup
Vanilla Yogurt & Fruit
Granola Cereal
Breakfast Trifle
French toast (eggy bread)
Breakfast muesli Smoothie
Creamy Oats with Maple syrup and Cinnamon
Dip Dip egg & Soldiers
Cheddar and Zucchini Breakfast muffins
Brekkie Wraps
100% Peanut butter on Wholemeal toast
Fruit kebabs
Mushroom and Cheese Omelette

Scrambled Eggs on Toast

Serves 2. Double up as needed.

Gold in an egg shell. Eggs are by far the best breakfast meal to feed the kids. Scrambled eggs take about the same time as the toast to cook. I have a non stick pan, so clean up is easy. I recommend investing in one of these if you haven't already.

Ingredients
    Fresh Eggs (2 per person)
    ¼ teaspoon organic butter
    Sea salt to taste
    OPTIONAL: Chopped chives or parsley to sprinkle on top
    Wholemeal toast

Instructions
Melt butter in a Non Stick Pan. Crack eggs into a bowl and whisk until well blended. Pour mix into a hot pan. Stir regularly until egg is cooked through. Serve with hot, buttered wholegrain toast.

NOTE from Carey: When I give this meal to my smaller kids (6 year old and 7 years old), I cut up the toast into bite sized squares and lay the egg on top. Kids are then able to use a knife and fork to easily eat their meal 'like a big kid' as they only need to cut the egg. My bigger kids started making scrambled eggs for themselves around 11yrs of age. It's a perfect 'first meal' for them to make on their own.

****

Wholemeal Banana Pancakes, Vanilla Yogurt & Maple Syrup

(Serves 6)

These little pancakes are always received with joy. They look a bit like 'junk food'' but contain about two serves of fruit per plate. I serve our pancakes in a three pancake stack with a layer of Vanilla Yogurt and sliced fruit between each layer. We then top it off with a drizzle of maple syrup and sprinkle of Cinnamon on top. My kids like sliced bananas, blue berries and strawberries best.

Ingredients
2 x ripe bananas mashed.
4 x eggs (slightly beaten)
2 cups Wholemeal Self Raising Flour
1 ½ cups of milk
½ teaspoon vanilla extract
Butter for frying

To Serve
100% maple syrup (warm slightly)
Vanilla Yogurt for Serving
Sliced banana or strawberries
Cinnamon

Instructions
Whisk eggs slightly. Add mashed banana, eggs, flour and milk. Mix together well with a hand mixer or whisk. Cover mix and allow to stand for 15-30 min. Heat up Pan and add a bit of butter to prevent pancakes sticking. Spoon approx 2 tablespoons of mixture per pancake into hot pan. I cook about 3 – 4 pancakes in a pan at a time. Turn when bubbles start to form on top of pancake.

Serve with Vanilla Yogurt, maple syrup and sliced bananas and a dash of cinnamon.

******

Vanilla Yogurt & Fruit

1 serve (double up as needed)

Vanilla yogurt is one of the most versatile recipes to know. When I refer to vanilla yogurt in any of my other recipes, this is the one I'm talking about. This recipe makes one serving, so double up as needed.

Ingredients
    1tablespoon maple syrup
    ½ cup of plain Greek Yogurt

Instructions
    Stir together until smooth. Serve chilled with fruit of your choice.

Note from Carey: When I first made this, I washed out a 'store bought' vanilla yogurt tub and remade my clean version inside. My two youngest didn't even notice the difference.

******

Granola Cereal

(makes12 serves)

Ingredients
Dry Ingredients:
   4 cups rolled raw oats
   1/2 cup chopped raw cashews
   1/2 cup chopped raw almonds
   ¼ cup chopped peanuts
   1/4 cup finely shredded raw coconut
   ½ cup raisin or dried fruit

Wet Ingredients:
   1/4 cup melted butter
   1 teaspoon vanilla extract
   1 cup honey

Instructions
Preheat oven to 250 degrees F (120 degrees C). Mix dry ingredients together. Mix wet ingredients together and then add to dry ingredient mix. Spread onto a baking tray. Bake for around 45-50 min. Stir every 15 min to make sure it cooks evenly all over. Turn off oven and allow to cool in oven.

   Cool granola completely before storing in an air-tight container.

******

Breakfast Trifle

Presentation is everything with this breakfast dish. I use short whiskey glasses (yes, this is why I buy them) and layer my trifle so that the kids can see the layers clearly. I like to make a thin layer of each so I can fit two layers of each ingredient into the glass, but if time is an issue, just one serving of each does the trick. If you have a bit more time in the morning, let the kids layer their own trifle.

Ingredients
    Clean Granola (see previous recipe:)
    Sliced fruit – We like bananas and strawberries
    Vanilla Yogurt (see recipe on page:)
    Optional – sprinkling of maple syrup and cinnamon

Instructions
Layer 1 Sliced fruit layer at bottom of the glass. Layer 2 Add a large spoon of yogurt. Layer 3 granola. Repeat if required. Optional - Sprinkling of maple syrup to finish. Serve with a long teaspoon (just because it looks cool).

******

French toast (Eggy bread)

Serves 2

Makes two slices of French toast, which serves 1 person in our family or two little kids. Double up as needed.

Ingredients
2 thick slices of 100% Whole grain / Rye or Whole grain bread
2 eggs (whisked)
Teaspoon butter
Maple Syrup
½ banana
Cinnamon

Instructions
Melt butter in pan .Put bread into egg mixture and turn until egg is soaked into both sides of the bread. Place eggy bread in pan and cook for around 1-1.5min or until side is golden brown. Turn and cook the other side. Serve immediately with sliced banana, drizzle of maple syrup and a sprinkle of cinnamon.

******

Breakfast Muesli Smoothie
Serves 1

Ingredients
1 banana
¼ cup natural muesli
2 -4 strawberries (frozen, fresh or dried are all good)
2 Tablespoons vanilla yogurt
¼ cup ice
¼ cup almond milk (or standard milk)

Instructions:
Blend all together until ice is properly crushed. Serve immediately. Add more almond milk if you don't like it too thick.
Note from Carey: I freeze Vanilla yogurt and pureed fruit in ice cube trays especially for smoothies. Each cube is approx 1 tablespoon.

Creamy Oats with Maple syrup and Cinnamon

So fast and easy plus it keeps kids tummy's nice and full too.

Ingredients
¼ cup dried oats (I use quick cook, organic oats which just means oats that have been chopped up a bit in the processor to make it quicker to cook and a bit smoother for kids to eat).
¼ cup boiling water
¼ cup heated milk / almond milk

Instructions:
Add boiled water and heated milk to oats. Cover and leave for approx two minutes. Stir. Add more milk if too thick. Serve with a sprinkle of cinnamon, sliced banana and swirl of maple syrup.

******

Dip Dip Egg & Soldiers

My grandmother would give this to us when all the cousins were sent to her during school holidays. I don't know how she did it, but she managed to serve up massive amounts of perfectly soft boiled eggs every time. 'Dip Dip eggs and soldiers' was a name thought up by one of us when we were young and it kinda just stuck.She even went the extra mile and sewed little elf hats (triangle felt pieces) for each of us. They slipped over our eggs, and we were allowed to draw pencil faces on our eggs while they cooled. When my children were little, I could add sliced celery, carrots and cucumber and they would happily dip these into their egg, but now that they are bigger, only buttered toast will do. TIP: if you add a small pinch of salt to the water it will help to stop the eggs cracking.

Ingredients
Soft boiled eggs (1 or two per person)
Rye / Wholemeal Toast – buttered and sliced into 1.5 cm strips (1 or two slices per person)

Instructions
How to make Soft Boiled Eggs: For us, a perfect soft boiled egg means adding a room temperature egg to a pot of boiling water (use a spoon to drop the egg SLOWLY into water to stop cracking) and simmer for 4 min exactly. When you find the time that works for you, write it down and keep it close. Perfectly boiled eggs are a work of art and closely guarded family secret). Serve soft boiled egg in an egg cup with buttered toast pieces..

FUN STUFF: For a little fun project, visit my website to download templates for easy egg warmer hats. You can find them here at www.cleaneatingwithkids.com/egghats

******

Cheddar and Zucchini Breakfast muffins

Makes 12 muffins

This recipe is a modification of a recipe I found on Allrecipes.com. made by Pam-"3BoysMama. Don't be put off by the Zucchini. They are delicious!

Ingredients
 1 and 1/2 cups wholemeal self raising flour (or if using plain flour, add 1.5 teaspoons of baking powder to plain flour)
 1/4 cup butter (melted)
 2 eggs (lightly beaten)
 1 cup milk
 1 cup zucchini (shredded unpeeled)
 3/4 cup shredded cheddar cheese
 1/4 cup grated Parmesan cheese (freshly)
 4 slices free range bacon (cooked crisp and diced into little bits)

Instructions
Preheat oven to 350 degrees F (175 degrees C). Grease 12 hole muffin tray with butter. Mix the flour and salt in bowl. In another bowl, stir together the butter, egg, milk, zucchini until well blended. Slowly add the flour mixture into the milk mixture and stir slowly until smoothly blended. Fold in the Cheddar cheese, Parmesan cheese, and crumbled bacon, and spoon the batter into the prepared muffin cups. Bake in the preheated oven for 20 to 25 minutes until tops are golden brown. Allow muffins to cool slightly before removing from muffin cups; serve warm. Refrigerate leftovers for tomorrow.

******

Brekkie Wraps

Serves 1. Increase quantities as needed.

Sunday morning breakfasts are normally a bacon and egg 'fry up'. I am not a fan of dirty eggy dishes, so Brekkie Wraps are my solution to this. By wrapping the egg and bacon in a wholegrain wrap, the meal is less of a fuss. Plus, if we need to eat on the run, I can easily wrap them up in foil for an on the go breakfast at the beach or weekend school sport event.

Ingredients:
1x Organic Rye Wraps or Wholegrain tortillas
1 x egg
1 x Rasher of free range bacon (shredded)
½ x banana (sliced longways through middle)
3 x button mushrooms – sliced

Instructions
Grease non stick frying pan with a bit of butter and heat up pan on stove. Shallow fry bacon and set aside. In same pan, fry mushrooms then banana until golden on both sides. To fry eggs: crack egg into pan. Once white has set on bottom, turn the egg to cook the white on top. Remove as soon as white is cooked, and egg still feels soft in middle. Place egg, bacon, mushrooms and banana in centre of wrap and roll up.

******

100% Peanut butter on Wholemeal toast

OK, so this is a bit self explanatory, but I had to add it in as it has to be one of the yummiest, fastest breakfasts available for those crazy school mornings. And you can even eat it in the car (if you have to).

The quality of peanut butter is what makes this special. Many supermarkets now sell an organic peanut butter made from *ONLY ONE* ingredient – peanuts. That's the one you are after. I buy this in bulk and use it in a lot of my recipes. Feel free to make up your own batch of peanut butter. I use the store bought organic version because, well to be honest, it's easier.

Ingredients
> Organic Peanut butter
> Wholegrain / Rye Bread.

Instructions
> Toast bread and spread thick with peanut butter. Cut toast into 4 easy to hold strips for kids and serve immediately.

NOTE from Carey: Read the ingredients list on the peanut butter. It should say 100% peanuts. That's it. Nothing else added.

****

Fruit kebabs

Serving size: 2 kebabs per person.

These are quick and easy to make for breakfast, after school snacks, dessert or even party food. They look amazing and are good for you too.

Ingredients
Slice up fruit into large ½ inch cubes/slices: Our favourites are banana, apple slices, watermelon, melon, kiwi fruit, grapes and strawberries. Wooden skewers

Instructions
Thread fruit onto a wooden skewer. Serve with yogurt dip on the side.

******

Mushroom and Cheese Omelette

Serves 1 adult or big kid (or two little kids). Increase quantities as needed.

I recommend investing in a good non-stick pan for this recipe, well worth it as these will become a regular part of your Clean Eating meal plan.

Ingredients:
2 eggs
Grated cheese

Filling options
Mushrooms - sliced and fried
Bananas - sliced and fried
Free range bacon - diced and fried
Onion - finely sliced and fried

Instructions:
Heat up your non stick pan over medium heat. Add a little bit of butter to prevent sticking. Whisk up eggs and pour into pan. Move the pan around to spread the egg over the bottom of the pan (like making an eggy pancake). The omelette will start to cook and firm up. Sprinkle cheese and cooked mushrooms (plus your choice of filling) on the top of the omelette. The top will still be a bit raw at this point. Use a spatula to fold the omelette in half. Cook a bit more until the omelette is golden underneath and cooked through. Slide onto plate and serve.

****

10 LUNCH TIME RECIPES

Tuna Rye Wraps
Salmon Patties
Mixed Veggie Slice
Spinach and Feta Muffins
Potato Wedges & Sour Cream
Macaroni and cheese
Cous Cous Salad
Chinese (not fried) rice
Mini Quiche
Wholemeal Pasta Salad

Tuna Rye Wraps

Serves 6

Ingredients
6 Wholegrain wraps or tortillas
2 tins of tuna in water
2 cups shredded lettuce
1 cup grated carrot
½ an onion – diced into very small pieces (OPTIONAL)
¼ cup Mayonnaise (I purchase an organic, store bought version from our Supermarket, but it's easy to make too. See Recipe on Pg 136.

Instructions:
Mix Tuna, Mayonnaise and onion together until well mixed and tuna chunks broken up. Combine lettuce and carrot in a mixing bowl. Place a 1/3 cup lettuce and carrot mix in a line down centre of wrap. Top with tuna. Roll up, cut in half and serve.

****

Salmon Patties

Serves 4 (makes 8 patties)

Ingredients
1 large sweet potato cooked and mashed
1 can 480g Salmon (OR two small 225g cans) drained and flaked. Remove any bones.
1 egg
1 teaspoon grated lemon rind
½ cup wholemeal flour
Salt and pepper

Instructions
Mix all ingredients together using your hands. Shape into walnut sized balls and flatten into hot pan.
Heat a frying pan on medium heat. Add sprinkle of olive oil to prevent sticking. Cook for about 3 minutes or until golden brown, turn and cook the other side.

Serve with a salad and lemon yogurt dip (see Pg 136).

****

Healthy Veggie Slice

Serves 6

Super easy way to use up any leftover vegetables. Tastes great and it is also perfect for lunch boxes or weekend picnics.

Ingredients
    1 onion finely diced
    ½ cup thinly sliced mushrooms
    250g cottage cheese
    3 eggs beaten
    1 cup wholemeal self raising flour
    1 cup grated vegetables: carrots, zucchini, corn kernels, spring onions, grated cabbage, cooked sweet potato, cooked pumpkin.
    1 cup finely chopped spinach
    ½ cup grated cheese
    ½ tablespoon melted butter

Instructions
Preheat oven to 180 degrees Celsius (or 350 degrees Fahrenheit) Grease a 2 litre oven dish. In a frying pan, heat butter and fry onion until soft (about 5 min). Add mushrooms. Fry for 2 more minutes until mushrooms are soft. In a mixing bowl, mix together cottage cheese and egg. Add flour, whilst mixing to prevent lumps. Stir through all remaining ingredients until combined. Pour into greased dish and Bake for 40-45min until golden. Cut into slices and serve. Can be served hot or cold

****

Spinach and Feta Muffins

Makes 12 large muffins

Ingredients

> 2 cups wholemeal self-raising flour
> 250g spinach (about 1/2 bunch) spinach, trimmed, washed, dried, shredded
> ¼ cup feta cheese, crumbled
> ½ cup grated cheddar cheese
> 330ml(1 1/3 cups) milk
> ¼ cup melted butter
> 2 eggs
> 1 tablespoon thinly sliced spring onions.

Instructions
Preheat oven to 180 degrees Celsius (or 350 degrees Fahrenheit)
Stir flour, cheese, spring onions and spinach together. Whisk eggs. Add eggs, butter and milk to flour mix. Stir until just combined. Spoon into greased muffin tray (12 hole tray or mini 24 hole tray). Bake for 15 minutes until golden brown.

Note: you can use frozen spinach for this recipe too. Allow frozen spinach to thaw and squeeze out excess water before using in recipe as above.

****

Oven Baked Potato Wedges with Sour Cream and Guacamole

(Serves 4-6)

Ingredients:
4 large potatoes - cut length ways into wedges (you can peel if you want, but it is OK to leave the peel on washed potatoes).
2 tablespoons olive oil
1 teaspoon dried rosemary.
Sea salt

Instructions
Preheat oven to 190 degrees Celsius (or 380 degrees Fahrenheit). Mix potatoes with salt, rosemary and oil until well coated. Place on oven tray and pop into hot oven for about 30 minutes. Potatoes will be golden brown and crispy on the outside. To check if they are cooked - break a wedge open. Potato will be soft inside.

Serve with Guacamole, salsa and Sour Cream on the side.

****

Macaroni and cheese

Serves 6 – 8

This meal on its own doesn't have vegetables in it, so I always serve it with a salad. It's great for school lunches too and my kids seem to love it hot or cold. I added it to my dinner list because it is simple to make and replaces those horrible store bought 'mac n cheese' boxes. I think it takes about the same amount of time to make too. Except – it's clean!

Ingredients
1 bag (500g) of wholegrain macaroni pasta (makes about 6 cups of cooked macaroni)
100grams of butter
½ cup of plain flour
3 cups of milk
¾ cup organic cheddar cheese
Sea Salt to taste

Instructions
Boil macaroni for around 8 minutes or until just undercooked. Macaroni should be a 'bit chewy'. Set aside in large oven proof bowl.

Cheese Sauce: Turn your stove top on to a medium heat. Melt butter is in a large, clean saucepan. Add flour and stir with a wooden spoon. The flour and butter will clump together like a ball of 'dough'. Start adding the milk ½ cup at a time and stir until smooth. The paste will thicken and lump. DO NOT add more milk until the lumps have been stirred out. Continue adding the milk ½ cup at a time until your sauce starts to take on a thick, saucy appearance. You can add more milk to thin out the mixture. Bring to a simmer, then remove the pot from the heat and add the cheese. Stir slowly until it melts into the sauce. Add salt to taste.

Preheat oven grill. Pour the sauce over the macaroni and mix through. Sprinkle ½ cup cheese on top, and place under grill. Grill until the top of the macaroni cheese is golden brown. Serve hot or cold with salad on the side.

Cous Cous Salad

Ingredients
- 1 ½ cups dry cous cous
- 2 spring onions – finely sliced
- 1 red pepper – finely diced
- ½ cup of cucumber – finely diced
- 1 cup of butternut pumpkin (diced)
- ¼ cup pine nuts
- 1 tablespoon olive oil

Instructions
Preheat oven to 400'F. Place butternut and pine nuts on oven tray and drizzle with olive oil. Bake for 15 minutes or until butternut is cooked through. While butternut is cooking, put dry cous cous into a large bowl and pour boiling water over it until water level is just above the cous cous (about 1/4 inch). Cover bowl, so that cous cous can absorb the water. Once all water is absorbed, use a fork to 'fluff' up the cous cous. This separates the grains so that they are not stuck together.

Add cooked pumpkin, pine nuts and all other ingredients to cooked cous cous and stir through. Serve warm or cold.

****

Chinese (not fried) rice

Serves 4-6

Kids will love this rice dish, and it's perfect for lunch boxes too!

Ingredients
1/2 carrot - grated
1/2 celery stick - diced
1/2 small red or green capsicum - seeds removed and diced
2 spring onions - sliced fine
1 can pineapple rings in natural or unsweetened juice - finely chopped. Set juice aside for dressing.
4 cups cooked and cooled basmati rice
4 tbs sweet corn kernels
OPTIONAL: Finely sliced bacon / ham or chicken pieces.

Dressing
1/4 cup Pineapple Juice
2 tablespoons tamari sauce

Instructions
Place all ingredients in mixing bowl
Using a spoon, mix thoroughly. If not using at once, cover with cling wrap (or transfer to a storage container) and refrigerate until needed.

NOTE: Tamari Sauce is not entirely clean, but is a healthy lower sodium substitute for Soy Sauce. I use it in small quantities in my stir fries and Asian dishes.

****

Mini Cheese and Bacon Quiche

Makes 12

This is an easy dish to make for breakfast, lunch and even a light dinner. You can add any vegetables or leftover meat to your quiches. I have a few of our favourite variations below.

Ingredients
- 4 whole grain wraps (cut into quarters)
- 1 Tablespoon butter
- 1 small onion - finely diced
- 4 rashers of free range bacon - finely chopped
- 6 eggs
- 1/2 cup grated cheese

Instructions
Preheat oven to 180 degrees Celsius (350 degrees Fahrenheit). Grease your 12 hole muffin tray with butter. Line each hole with one piece of the quartered Whole grain wrap. Heat a pot on the stove. Add butter, onions and bacon and fry on medium heat until onion has softened. Spoon the bacon and onion mix evenly on top of the wholegrain wraps. Whisk eggs until well blended. Divide evenly between quiches. Sprinkle cheese on top of each and place in the oven. Cook for about 12-15 minutes or until cheese is golden brown and egg is cooked through.

Here are a couple of ideas for Mini Quiche Variations. Simply add to the recipe or replace the bacon with any of the below ingredients:

Mushroom: 1 cup of finely sliced, cooked mushroom
Corn: 1 cup of cooked corn kernels
Feta and onion: 1/2 cup of crumbled feta
Ham and Cheese: 1/2 cup shredded ham
Asparagus: 3-4 chopped asparagus spears, lightly

NOTE: You can also use whole grain bread instead of wraps. You just need to flatten the bread with a rolling pin before using it.

****

Wholemeal Pasta Salad

Serves 4 -6

Ingredients
4 cups cooked wholemeal pasta (I like to use spirals or shell shapes)
1/2 cup diced cucumber
1/2 cup diced red pepper (capsicum)
1 can tuna (in water)
1/2 cup finely sliced celery
1/2 cup creamy lemon dressing

Creamy Lemon Dressing
1/4 cup plain Greek yogurt
2 tablespoons lemon juice
1 teaspoon honey
1 teaspoon Dijon mustard
Ground black pepper to taste
1 tablespoon olive oil
1 teaspoon chopped chives

Instructions:
Mix all dressing ingredients together and set aside.
Mix all salad ingredients together and add dressing when serving.

****

13 Busy Family Dinner Recipes

Beef Stroganoff
Creamy Chicken pie
Easy, Chicken Casserole
Beef Pot Roast, Potatoes and Gravy
Oven Baked Meatballs in tomato sauce and Spaghetti
Roast Chicken, Veg & Gravy
Hearty Crockpot Beef and Vegetable Stew
Clean Chicken Parmigiana
Creamy Fish Pie & peas
Smoked Fish Kedgeree
Spaghetti bolognaise
Fast Lasagne
Crockpot Chicken and Vegetable Soup

Beef Stroganoff

Serves 4-6

Ingredients
1 x onion diced
1 x tablespoon olive oil
800g Beef Strips
2 cups liquid vegetable stock
1 teaspoon onion powder
1 cup organic passata (tomato puree)
1 cup mushrooms - sliced
¼ cup sour cream

Instructions
Heat olive oil and onion in pan until onion is soft. Add beef strips and fry until meat is browned slightly. Add mushrooms and fry until softened. Add vegetable stock, onion powder, around ¼ teaspoon of salt and passata. Cook on medium heat for around half an hour until juices have reduced about two thirds of original amount and beef strips are tender. Remove from heat and stir in sour cream.

Serve with brown rice and peas.

****

Creamy Chicken pie

(Serves 6-8)

This lovely pie recipe is based on a Jamie Oliver Chicken and Leek Pie. I had to make a couple of changes as for some reason; my smaller children find the taste of thyme a bit too much to handle in large quantities. This changes as they get a bit bigger – don't ask me why. This is a great way to introduce leaks to your family. On their own they are a bit boring, but in this recipe, they just come together in a smooth, beautifully flavoured pie that even the fussiest of my children loves.

Wholemeal Pie Pastry: Ingredients:
    1 ½ cups whole wheat pastry flour
    ½ teaspoon salt
    ¼ cup butter
    ¼ cup COLD water
    1 egg

Pie Filling: Ingredients
    1tablespoon olive oil
    2 x large leeks sliced into 1cm wide circles
    4 x chicken breasts sliced into 1cm wide strips
    1 onion diced small
    4 cups of chicken or vegetable stock
    1 x teaspoon thyme leaves (dried of fresh)
    2 tablespoon flour
    ½ cup Greek yogurt or cream

Instructions
Wholemeal pastry. Rub the flour and salt together with the butter and until it has the texture of breadcrumbs, then work in the water and egg until a pastry comes together into a dough. Knead the pastry on a work surface until soft. Press the pastry into a flat round shape, then chill for 1 hr while you make the filling.

Filling: In a large saucepan, add onions and olive oil. Fry for around 5 min until onions have softened. Add chicken and cook until juices have evaporated and chicken slightly browned. Add leeks and thyme, cover pot and cook until leeks soften. Stir in the flour. Filling will thicken instantly. Add Stock and allow to simmer for around 20 minutes or until sauce has thickened to your liking. Remove from heat and stir through yogurt (or cream).

Place the filling into an oven proof dish and top with wholemeal pastry and Bake in preheated oven at 180 degrees Celsius (or 350 degrees Fahrenheit) for around 15 - 20 minutes or until pastry is golden and crispy.

Serve with mash potato and baby peas

****

Easy, Chicken Casserole

(Serves 4 –6)

This recipe can be doubled up, so I always try to make a double batch and pop one in the freezer for those days when crazy happens.

Ingredients

- 1 x tablespoon olive oil
- 6 x chicken thighs (filleted and sliced into 2cm strips)
- 1 x onion diced
- 1 x sliced garlic glove
- 4 cups of chicken or vegetable stock
- 2 medium potatoes (cubed into 2cm pieces)
- 1 medium sweet potato OR 1 cup diced pumpkin
- 2 thickly sliced carrots (1cm slices)
- ¼ cup tomato puree or passata
- Salt and Pepper to taste

Instructions

In a large saucepan, heat oil. Add diced onion and cook until softened (around 5 min). Add Sliced garlic and chicken strips. Cook chicken until juices have evaporated and chicken starts to brown slightly. Pour in Stock and tomato puree and simmer for around 20 minutes. Add vegetables and cook for a further 20 min until vegetables have softened. If you prefer a thicker consistency to your sauce, then thicken by stirring through 1 tablespoon of flour and cold water paste. (Mix flour and water until a smooth paste is formed and stir through the casserole, stirring the entire time. Sauce with thicken instantly. Season with salt and ground black pepper.

Serve with fluffy basmati rice or wholegrain pasta.

******

Beef Pot Roast, Perfect potatoes and bucket loads of thick, tasty gravy

Serves 6- 8

I cannot begin to tell you how good this meal is. There is something about a slow cooked roast, with a generous smothering of thick gravy that make everything just seem right. This pot roast is just as delicious the next day on sandwiches or simply reheated and enjoyed again.

Ingredients
1kg topside beef roast
½ teaspoon onion powder
1 kg potatoes (approx 5-6 potatoes) peeled and halved
1 litre of vegetable stock
¼ cup plain flour
½ cup COLD water
Tablespoon olive oil

Instructions
Heat up large, deep sided pot until hot! Add the Topside to the pot and Brown the pot roast completely all over. Keep turning until all sides have been browned. Do not let it burn. This shallow frying step is absolutely vital. It is a little secret that takes this meal from blah to wow – DO NOT SKIP THIS STEP. It will take about 5 minutes to do properly.

When you have sealed the roast all over, add your vegetable stock and onion powder to the pot. Turn down the heat and simmer for approx 1 hr. Add the potatoes to the sauce and let them boil in the same pot (or slow cooker). They will turn slightly brown on the outside as they soak up the flavour. Cook until potatoes soften, remove Meat and potatoes from sauce (which will appear very watery still) and set aside. Slice meat into thin slices.

NOTE: You may want to transfer to a slow cooker after you have added the vegetable stock. Allow to cook in slow cooker for around 2.5hrs.

How to Make Perfect Gravy

It's time to thicken up the sauce to make the gravy. In a cup, mix the flour with ¼ cup of <u>COLD</u> water until a smooth paste is formed. Bring the pot to the boil then remove from the heat and stir through the flour mixture. The gravy will thicken instantly. Add water if you don't want it too thick. Add the sliced beef and potatoes back to the gravy and let them soak in the flavour for a few minutes before serving.

Serve with brown rice and a steamed green beans, peas or broccoli.

******

Oven Baked Meatballs in tomato sauce (with hidden veg) and wholegrain spaghetti

Serves 6

This is one of my children's favourite meals. It's quick to prepare, and you can get it in the oven in around 10 min flat. This is my clean cheat meal. I use store bought organic tomato pasta sauce. Most Supermarkets now stock these options. Just remember to read through the ingredients: We want to see tomato, onion, garlic, herbs (that's it!).

Ingredients:
500g minced beef OR chicken.
2 Bottles of Organic Pasta Sauce (about 3 cups)
½ cup grated carrot
½ cup grated zucchini
1 egg
¼ teaspoon salt
2 teaspoons tomato paste
2 tablespoons plain organic flour
Wholemeal spaghetti

Instructions
Pre heat oven to 180 degrees Celsius (or 350 degrees Fahrenheit). In a large oven proof dish, pour both bottles of tomato pasta sauce, grated veggies. Set aside ready for meatballs. Meatballs: mix together minced meat, raw egg, tomato puree, salt and flour. Form tablespoon sized meat balls. Put the RAW meat balls into the sauce. Do not stir as the meatballs will break apart. Add all meatballs to sauce – looks a bit odd, but trust me here, it works! Bake UNCOVERED in oven for 30-40 min. Meatballs will be firm, browned slightly on top & sauce will be a thicker, rich red colour. Spoon meatballs and sauce onto cooked wholemeal pasta. Kids won't even know that they are eating tomato, carrots and zucchini – all in one dish!Serve with a fresh salad on the side.

NOTE: This recipe also works well in slow cooker, but seems to taste better when oven baked. Don't know why.

Roast Chicken, Veg & Gravy

(Serves 6)

Nothing - And I do mean NOTHING beats a Roast Chicken Dinner. Walking into a home that has a chicken slow roasting in the oven is almost heavenly.

Ingredients:
1 x Large Free Range Whole Chicken
4 x large potatoes quartered
2 x large sweet potatoes quartered
2 x cups chicken stock
¼ cup flour mixed with ½ cup COLD water

Chicken Rub Mix:
¼ teaspoon salt
2 tablespoons of olive oil
¼ teaspoon garlic powder
¼ teaspoon onion powder
¼ teaspoon dried rosemary

Instructions:

Preheat oven to 180 degrees Celsius (or 350 degrees Fahrenheit) Mix all Chicken rub ingredients together – rub all over raw chicken. Place chicken in LARGE metal oven tray. Baked uncovered for 30 – 40 min. Chicken should be smelling good, browning slightly but still undercooked.

Place potatoes into tray with chicken and bake for another 30 min or until potatoes are cooked through and crispy. Turn once during cooking. Check Chicken is cooked and juices running clear (otherwise leave for a bit longer). Remove Chicken and potatoes from pan and set aside.

The Best Ever Roast Chicken Gravy

In the same pan that you cooked the chicken. Stir in the chicken stock and flour and water mix. Place on stove top and heat. Keep stirring until sauce thickens and begins to simmer.

Remove from heat and pour into gravy jug.

To Serve: Carve up chicken into serving size pieces. Serve with brown rice, Roast potatoes and fresh vegetable and gravy. I like to add corn and broccoli to our plates – just because it looks beautiful.

******

Hearty Crockpot Beef and Vegetable Stew

Serves 6-8

I added this recipe after watching my entire brood finish every bit on their plates. It's a budget meal that stretches a long, long way and it can easily stretch to two good sized meals for our family of six. The stew itself freezes beautifully, but I like to make a fresh batch of rice for each meal.

Ingredients:
    2kg of blade beef (sometimes called Y Bone)
    2 diced onions
    2 tablespoons of olive oil
    2 cloves crushed garlic
    1 litre of organic beef or vegetable stock
    4 large potatoes - quartered
    3 large carrots sliced into 1cm slices
    1 teaspoon onion powder
    4 tablespoons tomato paste
    ¼ cup plain flour
      ½ cup water
    Sea Salt to taste (Taste first, as Beef stock is often salty)

Instructions:
Add olive oil, onions, garlic and beef to a hot pot. Cook for around 5 min until onions have softened and juices have reduced. Stir through onion powder & tomato paste. Add Stock and simmer for around 40-50 min or until meat is tender. Add potatoes and carrots and simmer for an additional 20 min or until potatoes are cooked through.

In a cup: mix flour and water to a smooth paste. Stir quickly into stew. Sauce will thicken instantly. Allow to simmer for around 5 minutes. For a slightly creamier stew, you can remove from heat and stir through 2 tablespoons of cream or yogurt just before serving.

Note from Carey: Aadd more vegetables to this meal to keep it all in the one pot, but I like to serve with green beans on the side. Leftovers can be made into a beef pie – just add the wholemeal pastry on top.

Clean Chicken Parmigiana

Serves 4 – 6

The first time I made this was a mistake. I didn't read the recipe correctly and forgot to add breadcrumbs to my chicken. I had seen a picture in a magazine of the meal, but couldn't quite make out that the Chicken was coated in breadcrumbs. The short of it is, we ended up with a beautiful, healthy, whole food meal that is now a regular player in my monthly meal plan.

Ingredients
    1 tablespoon olive oil
    4 x chicken breasts cut in half length ways (8 thin pieces).
    2 bottles of clean tomato pasta sauce
    1/4 cup grated cheese
    8 x potatoes (peeled, boiled and mashed)

Instructions
Preheat Oven to 180 degrees Celsius (or 350 degrees Fahrenheit)
Heat oil in pan. Lightly brown chicken pieces turning once (doesn't have to cook through). Remove chicken from pan and lay in oven proof dish. Pour pasta sauce over chicken pieces to cover. Stir to coat chicken. Sprinkle cheese on top and place in oven for 115-20 minutes or until cheese is golden and chicken is cooked through.

Mashed Potatoes: Place potatoes in a large pot of boiling water and cook until potatoes soft. Drain water and mash together with 2 tablespoons of butter and 1/2 cup of milk. Season with salt and pepper. Set aside.
Serve with fresh broccoli or green beans.

NOTES: You can make pasta sauce from scratch, but I recommend finding a good quality pasta sauce at your local Supermarket. It will save you a heap of time and sanity in the kitchen. For those of you want to put in the extra effort, I have a recipe for Clean Pasta Sauce on my website at www.cleaneatingwithkids.com/pastasauce if you are interested.

****

Creamy Fish Pie

Serves 6-8

Ingredients:

  4 - 6 skinless smoked haddock fillet (or other smoked fish)
  2 1/2 cups full fat milk
  1 small onion, finely diced
  3 hard boiled eggs, chopped
  1 cup of frozen peas
  small bunch parsley, leaves only, chopped
  4 tablespoons of butter
  2 tablespoons plain flour
  6 large floury potato, peeled and cut into even-sized chunks
  1/2 cup cheddar, grated

Ingredients:

Preheat Oven to 180 degrees Celsius (or 350 degrees Fahrenheit) Place potatoes in a large pot of boiling water and cook until potatoes soft. Drain water and mash together with 2 tablespoons of butter and 1/2 cup of milk. Season with salt and pepper. Set aside. This will be your fish pie topping. In a large saucepan, place fish, onion and remaining 2 cups of milk. Bring to the boil and simmer for about 7-8min until fish starts to flake. Remove from heat. Remove fish and set milk aside to use later. Flake fish into bite sized pieces. To make the white sauce, melt 2 tablespoons of butter in a saucepan. Add flour to make a paste, then slowly add the milk (from earlier) at a rate of 1/4 cup at time. Stir consistently to avoid lumps forming. Remove from heat and stir in fish pieces, chopped eggs, parsley, frozen peas. Pour into an oven proof dish and spread mashed potato on top and sprinkle with grated cheese. Pop the fish pie into the hot oven and bake for 30 min. Cheese will be grilled and browned on top. Serve on its own or with a side salad

****

Smoked Fish Kedgeree

Serves 6

This is a good way to introduce your child to a curry. It has a 'curry taste', but no burn. Leftovers are perfect for school lunches as it is great served hot or cold.

Ingredients

3 cups cooked basmati rice.
3 hard boiled eggs. Sliced.
600g (2 large smoked fish fillets – I use smoked haddock) steamed or poached and broken into small pieces. Check that all bones are removed.
1 cup cooked vegetables (peas, beans, carrots)
1 tablespoon butter
1 onion finely diced
1 clove of garlic crushed.
2 tablespoon MILD curry powder
¼ cup coriander leaved chopped

Instructions:

Heat butter in pan. Add onions, garlic and curry powder. Cook until onions have softened. Add all remaining ingredients and stir through until heated and thoroughly mixed. Serve with a fresh cucumber salad. See Pg 148.

****

Spaghetti bolognaise

Serves 6-8

Kids love Spaghetti Bolognaise. It's a feel good dish that warms the tummy and satisfies the fussiest eater. This is my "What shall I cook" meal. On days when I don't feel like cooking, I generally have a serve of Spaghetti Sauce in my freezer. This recipe can easily be stretched across two meals (sometimes three). Divide into three portions and pop two into the freezer. It means two days of easy meals.

Ingredients
> 1 tablespoon olive oil
> 500g minced meat (beef or Chicken)
> 2 tablespoons tomato puree
> ¼ teaspoon salt
> 2 cups organic pasta sauce
> ½ cup grated carrot
> Cooked Wholemeal spaghetti

Instructions

Heat up pot on medium/high heat. Add oil, minced meat and salt. Fry until meat is dry and slightly browned. Add tomato puree and mix until mince well coated. Stir through pasta sauce & carrot (you can add additional veggies at this point to bulk up meal if needed). Turn heat down to low, cover and simmer for approx 20min. Serve on cooked Wholemeal pasta and Top with grated Parmesan cheese.

Serve with Italian Salad and Garlic Pita Bread

NOTE: If you have a few spare minutes on your hand and you really, truly don't have anything else you want to do. I know, I'm smiling while I type this, then head on over to my website to get the recipe for making your own pasta sauce from scratch. Here is the link: http://www.cleaneatingwithkids.com/pasta-sauce/

******

Fast Lasagne

Serves 6 – 8.

This is a fail proof dish which can be prepared, covered and placed in fridge/freezer for later. Just thaw and place in oven - Just like a 'bought one'. Keep leftovers in the fridge for tomorrow's lunch.

Ingredients
- 1 tablespoon olive oil
- 500g minced meat (beef OR chicken)
- 2 tablespoons tomato paste
- ¼ teaspoon salt
- 2 cups organic pasta sauce
- ½ cup grated carrot
- Uncooked wholemeal lasagne sheets
- 1 cup spinach leaves (optional)
- 1 cup grated cheese
- 2 cups milk
- ¼ cup plain flour
- ½ cup COLD water
- ½ teaspoon salt

Instructions
Pasta sauce: Heat up pot on medium/high heat. Add oil, minced meat and salt. Fry until meat is dry and slightly browned. Add tomato paste and mix until mince well coated. Stir through pasta sauce & carrot (you can add additional veggies at this point to bulk up meal if needed). Turn heat down to low, cover and simmer for approx 20min.

Quick White Sauce: Stir water and flour until smooth paste is formed. Add to cold milk. Heat up milk and flour mix in saucepan, stirring consistently. Sauce will start to thicken quickly when heated. Remove from heat once it comes to the boil. Stir through ¼ cup grated cheese.

Building your lasagne: In a large, oven proof dish spread out 1/3 of minced meat. Add a thin layer of spinach leaves, then a layer of lasagne sheets. Repeat until you have three layers. On top of third layer, pour white sauce and spread to cover. Sprinkle remaining grated cheese on top. (At this point, you can either continue to heat and eat, or cover and freeze for another day).

Bake in oven for 40min at 180 degrees Celsius (or 350 degrees Fahrenheit)

Slice into squares and serve with salad.

******

Crockpot Chicken and Vegetable Soup

Serves 8 – 10.

This dish can be made in one large pot on the stove, but the easy option is to use the crock pot. I pop it on at around lunchtime and it's perfect by dinner.

Ingredients:

1 tablespoon olive oil
6 x chicken thigh fillets (cut into 2 or 3 pieces each)
1 x large potato (peeled and cut into roughly 1 inch pieces)
1 x sweet potato (peeled and cut into roughly 1 inch pieces)
1 x large carrot (sliced into chunky slices)
1 cup pumpkin (peeled and cut into roughly 1 inch pieces)
2 x onions (diced)
1 head of broccoli (broken up)
½ cup of cream
1 litre (4 cups of Chicken or Vegetable Stock)

Instructions

Heat up Crockpot and add oil.
Add Chicken and onions and cook until juices have cooked away.
Add potatoes, sweet potatoes, pumpkin, carrot and stock.
Allow to boil for 2 hours on high.
Turn down to medium.
Add broccoli. Cook for an additional 20 minutes.
Mash the soup with a potato masher to break up any larger pieces of vegetable.
Turn off crock pot and add cream.
Serve with wholemeal bread (to dip)

Freezer Note: This dish freezes very well and reheats perfectly. Thaw overnight in the fridge and reheat in a pot on the stove.

******

6 Junk Food Recipes (with a Clean Twist)

Fish & Chips
Best Beef (or Chicken) Burgers
Cous Cous Chicken Nuggets and Oven baked Chips
Hot Chips
Pizza (Two Ingredient Pizza Dough)
Indian Butter Chicken
Quick Naan Bread / Flat bread wraps
Nachos

Fish & Chips

Serves 6

Who doesn't love fish and chips? This is a yummy dish but it has one important requirement: You MUST use FRESH fish. The Supermarket stuff just doesn't cut it. We are lucky to have a local fish shop selling fish right off the dock.

Ingredients

4 Firm White fish fillets (I normally use Hoki). Sliced into 1inch strips
2 eggs slightly beaten
1 cup plain flour
1 teaspoon onion powder
¼ teaspoon salt
4 tablespoons olive oil
8 Potatoes - cut into chip shapes wedges

Instructions

Chips: Preheat oven to 180 degrees Celsius (or 350 degrees Fahrenheit). Place potatoes on baking tray and mix together with salt and 2 tablespoons olive oil. Spread out on tray and place in hot oven. Bake for around 25minutes or until golden brown and crisp. Turn potatoes (shake up baking tray) about half way through cooking to crisp all sides.

Fish: Heat up non stick pan on medium heat. Add 1 tablespoon olive oil. Set up your ' fish station' next to the stove. In one bowl you have the beaten eggs. In another dish, mix together flour, salt and onion powder.

Take a strip of fish and dip into egg. Then dip into flour. Coat all sides. Add fish to hot pan. Cook in batches, turning until all sides are golden brown. Repeat until all fish is cooked. Lay on absorbent paper towel when done to soak up any excess oil.

Note from Carey: For that 'fast food' appeal, serve wrapped in Newspaper with Hot Oven Baked Chips, fresh lemon wedges and Tzatziki Dip. See page 137.

****

Best Beef (or Chicken) Burgers

Serves 6

Load up homemade burgers with fresh veggies or salad and you have a healthy meal that kids think is a real treat. I usually put all the ingredients on the table and let everyone create their own burger stack.

Ingredients

Burgers
500g minced meat (beef or Chicken)
1 teaspoon onion powder
1 tablespoons tomato puree
¼ cup plain flour
1 egg
¼ teaspoon salt
6 Wholegrain rolls
Organic BBQ Sauce / Organic Ketchup

Salad Filler (Any or all of these)
Lettuce – shredded
Tomato slices
Cheese – slices
Beetroot – boiled and finely sliced
Grated Carrot

Instructions
Beef Patties: Mix meat, onion powder, tomato puree, flour, egg and salt together. Shape into 6 round balls and flatten into patties.

Preheat pan or BBQ. Lighten coat each patty with a bit of olive oil and add to BBQ/pan. Cook each side for around 5 minutes. Meat should be browned and juices should run clear. Set aside and get your rolls ready.

Layer salad on rolls and top with beef patty and BBQ sauce. Serve immediately.

Note from Carey: Some things I just don't make from scratch. Frankly, I just draw the line at putting in the time and effort to make something that isn't going to end up being a complete meal. It's up to you – but my advice: "Choose your battles" and make it easy on yourself. BBQ sauce and tomato ketchup are two of those things. Organic versions of both are available from my local health store and now our local Supermarket.

Cous Cous Chicken Nuggets and Oven baked Chips

Serves 6

Ingredients

½ cup wholemeal cous cous
½ cup grated parmesan cheese
800g chicken breasts – sliced into 1cm strips
Pinch of salt
1 egg lightly beaten

Instructions

Preheat oven to 180 degrees Celsius (or 350 degrees Fahrenheit)
Place cous cous into heatproof bowl and add ½ cup boiling water. Cover and allow to stand for 5 min. Use a fork to 'fluff up' the cous cous grains and loosen them up. Allow to cool.
Mix parmesan cheese with cous cous, add a pinch of salt to season.
Dip chicken slices into egg and then roll in cous cous mixture. Press down a bit to make it stick.
Lay chicken in rows on oven tray and bake for around 20min or until golden. Turn occasionally until cooked through.

Serve with a side of oven baked chips.

****

Oven Baked Chips

Serves 4 -6

Ingredients

4 large potatoes – sliced length ways into 'chip' shape. You can use sweet potato or standard potatoes in this recipe.
Greased oven tray.
1 tablespoons olive oil
¼ teaspoon salt

Instructions

Preheat oven to 180 degrees Celsius (or 350 degrees Fahrenheit)
Use your hands to coat sliced potatoes with oil and salt.
Lay in a single layer on oven tray and pop into oven (with chicken nuggets)
Bake for 20-25min until chips are golden brown and crispy.

****

Pizza (with my Two Ingredient Pizza Dough)

Serves 4-6

Two Ingredients Pizza Base? YES! This Recipe has been shared over 35,000 times at the time I wrote this book. I use this for pizza bases, garlic pita bread and camping bread. I like to make mini pizza bases (around 10cm in diameter) as they fit perfectly into lunch boxes and kids get to add their toppings to their own pizzas.

Pizza Base Ingredients:
2 cups Wholemeal Self Raising Flour
200ml Greek Yogurt

Topping ideas:
Organic Pasta Sauce
Organic cheese (grated)
Mushrooms
Free Range Bacon
Pineapple
Banana
Spinach

Instructions:
Preheat oven to around 180 degrees Celsius (or 350 degrees Fahrenheit)
Knead flour and Greek yogurt together until you have a well mixed dough. Divide into 2 or 8 or 10 even balls (depends on the size pizza you want). Roll out with a rolling pin and ..... drum roll please .... your pizza bases are ready to go.
Spread Pasta Sauce on uncooked pasta base
Sprinkle Cheese and add Toppings
Bake in oven for around 10min.
Serve with a Fresh Salad on the side

To FREEZE: I like to have these ready to go, so stack bases on top of each other with baking paper between. Then wrap the stack in cling film and freeze. To thaw, simply remove and leave on bench top for around 5 min.

****

Indian Butter Chicken

Serves 6-8

This is a mild, delicious Indian Style curry that all my children love to eat. I wasn't going to include this recipe, as it takes a bit more effort than my usual meals, however ... it's a rainy day and as I write this, I have a huge pot cooking away on the stove. My home is filled with the most gorgeous aroma and kids are lining up to ask "when will dinner be ready, Mom?". I had to share.

Ingredients
    1kg chicken thigh fillets
    ¾ cup Greek yogurt (sour cream works well too)
    1 teaspoon ground ginger.
    2 cloves crushed garlic
    Juice of 1 lemon
    2 tablespoon olive oil
    ¼ cup coriander chopped
    3 tablespoons Garam Masala
    2 onions – thinly sliced
    1 tsp turmeric
    2 cups passata (tomato puree)
    1 cup cream
    ½ cup mint roughly chopped

Instructions

Marinade: Mix together: yogurt, ginger, garlic, lemon, olive oil, ½ the coriander, ½ the Garam Masala. Add the chicken thigh fillets and mix until thoroughly coated. Cover and leave in refrigerator for around two hours.

Preheat an oiled BBQ or char grill pan. Remove chicken from marinade and add each piece to the pan. Cook in batches until each piece of chicken is slightly grilled and almost cooked through (around 5 minutes)

In a large saucepan, add 1 tablespoon olive oil, onion, turmeric, remaining garam masala and cook until onions soften. Add chicken and passata, mint and remaining coriander. Cook on low for around 20 min. Stir occasionally. I like the chicken to be pulling apart slightly. Remove from heat and slowly stir in cream. Cook on low for 5 more minutes to thicken sauce.

Note from Carey: Prepare the chicken in the morning so that it can marinade for a couple of hours before you begin dinner.

Serve with Basmati Rice, Cucumber and Tomato salad (Sambal) and Quick Naan Bread.

****

Quick Naan Bread / Flat bread wraps

Makes 4

This is a versatile Naan bread recipe that can also double up as flat bread wraps.

Ingredients
2 cups plain flour. (Wholegrain is OK, but I use organic white flour for Naan bread and wholegrain when I am making flat bread wraps).
1 teaspoon yeast
½ cup warm water
½ warm milk
1 tablespoon olive oil or melted butter

Instructions

Mix together yeast, milk and water until yeast is dissolved. In a large mixing bowl, slowly add yeast mixture to flour, mixing as you go until soft ball of dough is formed. Cover bowl with dishcloth and set aside in a warm spot for around 15 minutes.

Knead the dough for around 3 minutes with your hands. Divide into four evenly sized balls. Using a rolling pin, roll each ball out until they flat – like a pancake. Move the dough around as you do this to prevent sticking.

Heat a non stick pan on medium/high heat. Add ½ tablespoon butter. Lay rolled dough in hot pan. Cook for around 30 seconds. Flip when golden, and cook the other side. Repeat with remaining naan pieces.

****

Nachos

Serves 6

Organic Plain Corn Tortillas are surprisingly clean. They are minimally processed with few ingredients. Read the ingredients list and opt for Tortillas with ingredients that you recognize.

Ingredients
250g Corn Tortilla Chips
1/2 cup grated Cheddar Cheese
1/4 cup diced Red Pepper (Capsicum)
¼ cup diced mushrooms
1 small red onion
1 tablespoon olive oil

Serve with
Sour Cream
Salsa
Guacamole

Instructions

Gently fry red pepper, onion and mushrooms in a pan until soft. Preheat oven to 180 degrees Celsius (or 350 degrees Fahrenheit). In a large oven tray, spread out Tortilla chips, sprinkle red pepper mix and cheese evenly on top.

Place in hot oven for around 5-8 minutes or until cheese starts to bubble. Serve with Sour Cream, Salsa and Guacamole on the side.

NOTE: You can use wholemeal wraps instead of tortillas. Slice up wraps into small triangle or squares and toast lightly in oven until they are crisp. Then use as in recipe above.

******

8 Dips & Dressings

Home Made Mayonnaise
Lemon Yogurt Dip
Cream Cheese and Chives Dip
Tzatziki Dip (Ziki Ziki Dip)
Simple Salsa
Guacamole
Italian Vinaigrette
Mango salsa

Home Made Mayonnaise

Makes about 2 cups of mayonnaise

Now in all honesty, I don't like making Mayonnaise. There are so many healthy options available at most Supermarkets, so I normally just buy it ready made. But, here is the recipe if you ever get stuck without it, and you have a (dressing deprived) tuna salad and guests arriving and shops are closed....

Ingredients:
4 fresh raw egg yolks
Pinch of salt
2/3 cup olive oil or milder-flavoured oil,
2/3 cup coconut oil (its sets hard at room temp, so this needs to be slightly melted to liquid)
1 Tablespoon lemon juice or apple cider vinegar
1 teaspoon of Dijon mustard

Instructions
Put egg yolks into blender or bowl and whisk/blend until smooth
Add lemon juice or vinegar, mustard and spices and blend until it well mixed.
SLOWLY add oil while blending or whisking at low speed, starting with olive oil. Start with a drop at a time until it starts to emulsify and then keep adding around a teaspoon at a time until the mayo has a creamy consistency.
Store in fridge up to 1 week.

NOTE: Homemade mayonnaise may separate, or "break," in the refrigerator. If needed, re-emulsify the mayo by stirring in a few droplets of water until it's nice and creamy again. Remember, this recipe contains RAW eggs, so throw away after 1 week if unused.

****

Lemon Yogurt Dip:

Mix together

1/4 cup plain Greek yogurt
2 tablespoons lemon juice
1 teaspoon honey
1 teaspoon Dijon mustard
Ground black pepper to taste
1 tablespoon olive oil
1 teaspoon chopped chives

******

Cream Cheese and Chives Dip

Mix together
½ cup cream cheese
¼ cup chopped chives.
2 tablespoons lemon juice

****

Tzatziki Dip
Makes 1 ½ cups

Mix together

1 cup of Greek yogurt
½ cup cucumber diced
½ clove garlic clove crushed
1 tablespoon of lemon juice.

****

Simple Salsa

This is a tasty addition to so many meals. When I think a dish is a bit 'dry', and I don't feel like making gravy, I make a batch of salsa to throw on top.

Mix together:

    2 large ripe tomatoes - finely diced
    1 small red onion - finely diced
    ¼ cup finely diced cucumber.
    Juice of 1/2 lemon (or lime)
    1 tablespoon balsamic vinegar

    OPTIONAL: 1/2 cup corn kernels

****

Guacomole

Serves 4-6

This recipe is perfect as a dip for crackers, corn tortillas and vegetable slices. It is important that your Avo's are ripe.

Ingredients:
    2 large RIPE Avocados - halved, peeled and stones removed
    1 small red onion - finely diced
    1 tomato - finely diced
    1 clove crushed garlic
    1/4 cup coriander - finely chopped
    Juice of 1 lime
    Salt and pepper to taste

Instructions.
Mix all ingredients together. Serve immediately.

******

Italian Vinaigrette

Ingredients

1/4 cup olive oil
1/2 teaspoon honey
3 tablespoon vinegar (white wine or balsamic)
1/2 teaspoon dried oregano (or fresh, chopped oregano)

Mix all ingredients together.

******

Mango salsa

Thank you to Michelle T. for sharing this little beauty of a salsa on my Facebook Page. We had a flood of Mangoes this season that, I swear, plotted to ripen on exactly the same day. I made this salsa up in bucket loads and served it on top of Grilled BBQ chicken. It was gorgeous!

Ingredients
½ cup Diced mango
½ cup Diced cucumber
1 small Diced red onion
2 Tbsp chopped fresh mint
2 Tbsp sweet chilli sauce or honey (I've tried both)

Mix all together and serve
You can have variations, such as diced red/yellow pepper or tomatoes also.

******

11 Salads & Vegetable Sides

Carrots with Honey and Sesame
Green Beans and Potato
Creamed Spinach
Curried Cabbage
Mash Potato Crunchies
Corn and Carrot Fritters
Cauliflower & Broccoli in Cheese sauce
Cucumber and tomato sambal (salad)
Carrot, Orange and Pineapple Salad
Cheese, tomato and cucumber stack

Honey Sesame Carrots

Serves 6

Ingredients:
6 carrots peeled and thinly sliced length ways
2 tablespoons of honey
1 teaspoon butter
1 tablespoon sesame seeds

Instructions
In a Saucepan, heat butter and lightly saute carrots for around 2 minutes. Add honey and sesame seeds to pan. Mix together. Serve.

****

Green Beans and Potato

Serves 4-6

When I was little, my grandmother was the bean growing master. I remember spending many an afternoon helping her pick, pack and freeze thousands of green beans. When it came to preparing them, there was only one recipe that all the grandkids ate. Here it is - I am happy to pass it on to you and your family.

Ingredients:
2 large potatoes, peeled, diced and boiled until soft (around 8 minutes)
250g green beans (washed, ends trimmed and sliced into 1cm pieces)
1 onion finely diced.
2 tablespoons butter
Salt and pepper to taste

Instructions
In a Saucepan, heat butter and lightly sauté onions until soft. Add beans and cook for 2 minutes to soften slightly. Add cooked potato pieces to pan and stir through until beans and potato are thoroughly mixed (The potato will mash up a bit). Season to taste and serve.

****

Creamed Spinach

Serves 4-6

This one will have your kids asking for more. It is a bit decadent for a vegetable side, but well worth the effort.

Ingredients:

1 large bunch of Spinach washed and finely sliced (approx 400g)
2 small onions - finely diced
2 garlic cloves crushed
2 tablespoons butter
200g creamed cheese (cut into small cubes)
1/2 cup milk

Instructions

In a large saucepan, heat butter over medium. Add onion and garlic. Cook, stirring occasionally, until onion softens (3 to 5 minutes). Add sliced spinach and sauté until all liquid evaporated and spinach has wilted. Stir through creamed cheese and milk. Creamed cheese will melt on heating. Keep stirring until well mixed. Serve immediately.

****

Curried Cabbage

Serves 4-6

A South African recipe that adds an interesting spin on regular ol' cabbage.

Ingredients:

Half a cabbage - washed and finely shredded
2 small onions - finely diced
2 garlic cloves crushed
2 tablespoons butter
1 tablespoons of mild curry powder (for a VERY mild curry flavour, skip the curry powder and replace with 1 tablespoon of garam masala. It has no heat, but does give a curry taste)

Instructions

In a large saucepan, heat butter over medium. Add onion and garlic. Cook, stirring occasionally, until onion softens (3 to 5 minutes). Add sliced spinach and saute until all liquid evaporated and spinach has wilted. Stir through creamed cheese and milk. Creamed cheese will melt on heating. Keep stirring until well mixed. Serve immediately.

****

Mash Potato Crunchies

Serves 8-12

My kids love this recipe. If you enjoy crispy roast potatoes, then I recommend you give this recipe a go. It will become a regular in your kitchen. I use a 12 hole muffin tray and full each hole to around half so that serving sizes are not too big. It looks a bit fancy, but it is just as easy as making standard mash potato, except that you pop it in the oven for the final step. You can add more vegetables in your potato mix such as peas, corn and carrots to make an all in one vegetable side.

Ingredients:

3 cups of mashed potatoes
1/2 cup sour cream
1/4 cup grated cheddar cheese
2 tablespoons butter
1/4 cup sliced chives or spring onion
Salt and pepper to taste

Instructions

In a large bowl, mix all ingredients together. Grease your muffin tray with some butter and spoon mixture evenly into each muffin hole (Amount will depend on how large you want your serving size to be). Bake at 400'F / 180'C for 30-35 minutes or until potato is golden and crunchy.

****

Corn and Carrot Fritters

Makes 14

I got this recipe from a friend after my children ate a small mountain of them at her home. I don't think they knew what was inside them. These fritters make a really delicious lunch time snack and work well in school lunch boxes too.

Ingredients

2 eggs, lightly beaten
2 cups wholemeal self raising flour
2 cups raw grated vegetables: carrots, zucchini, corn kernels, spring onions, grated cabbage.
1 cup grated cheese
40g butter

Instructions

Fold flour, vegetables and cheese into beaten eggs.
Grease non stick pan with butter and heat on medium heat.
Use ¼ cup scoop to pour mix into pan. I cook 3 at a time.
Cook until golden on both sides, flipping when done.

Serve with Salad, or own or with a Cream cheese or Tzatziki dip

****

Cauliflower and Broccoli in Cheese Sauce

Serves 6

Ingredients:

1/2 head cauliflower washed and broken into pieces
1 med - large broccoli washed and broken into pieces
1/2 cup grated cheddar cheese
2 tablespoons Parmesan Cheese.
2 cups milk
1/4 cup plain flour
2 tablespoons butter

Instructions

Preheat oven to 180 degrees Celsius (or 350 degrees Fahrenheit). Briefly boil or steam the broccoli and cauliflower for around 5 minutes. Veggies will still be a quite crisp. Drain and set aside. Place a large pan on the stove, melt butter and stir in flour. Slowly add milk, about 1/4 of a cup at a time, stirring continuously until all the milk is used. Remove from heat and stir in the Parmesan. Place broccoli and cauliflower in an oven proof dish and pour the sauce over. Sprinkle with cheese and bake for about 15 minutes until cheese is golden on top.

****

Cucumber and tomato sambal (salad)

Ingredients

1 cup diced tomato
1 cup diced cucumber
1 onion diced (optional)
¼ cup chopped mint
1 tablespoon lemon juice
1 tablespoon balsamic vinegar
1 tsp olive oil

Instructions

Mix all ingredients together. Keep covered in fridge for up to 48 hours.

****

Carrot, Orange & Pineapple Salad
Serves 4-6

This is a salad that screams Summer. It's gorgeous and I dare you to find a child that won't eat it.

Ingredients:
4 large carrots - peeled and grated
1/2 pineapple - peeled and finely diced (OR 1 can of pineapple in own juice)
Juice of two freshly squeezed oranges

Instructions

Mix all ingredients together. Refrigerate until ready to serve.

****

Cheese, Tomato and Cucumber stack

Serves 4-6

A simple salad stack changes up the presentation of your usual salad. It is still the same ingredients, but … stacked. You can use any salad ingredients, but I generally stick to these three - tomato, cheese and cucumber - They work really well together and I always have them in my fridge.

Ingredients:

1/2 cucumber - sliced into circles
2 tomatoes - sliced into circles
Cheese - finely sliced (I use a vegetable peeler to get my cheese sliced nice and thin.
Italian Vinaigrette

Instructions

On each plate, build a stack of cucumber, tomato and cheese - alternating each layer. I build up about 2 - 3 layers of each (it depends on how thick my slices are - and gravity, of course :)
Drizzle your Vinaigrette over the stack. Serve.

****

Easy Potato Salad

Serves 4-6

We have now arrived at my favourite salad. When I was pregnant, I devoured enough potato salad to feed a small nation. It is seriously yummy.

Ingredients:

4 large potatoes -peeled, diced and boiled
4 hard boiled eggs - peeled and diced.
125 ml sour cream
125 ml Greek yogurt
1 bunch fresh chives, finely sliced
2 stalks of celery – finely sliced
Salt and pepper to taste
OPTIONAL: 1 teaspoon wholegrain Dijon mustard (for a bit of a stronger taste)

Instructions

Mix all ingredients together. Refrigerate for about an hour before serving.

****

9 Clean Anytime Snacks

Banana Bread
No Lumps Apple & Cinnamon Muffins.
Carrot Cake
Granola bars (or Breakfast Granola)
Easy Peanut Butter Biscuits
Quick Cheese "Quackers"
Simply Yum Chocolate Biscuits
Popcorn 3 ways
Tapas

Banana Bread

(Makes 1 loaf or 12 medium sized muffins)

Never waste those over ripe bananas again. Learn this recipe by heart and you will be able to whip it up whilst washing up after dinner. Fresh banana bread for school lunches ready for the morning and you will be Mommy-of-the-year.!

Ingredients

3 over ripe mashed bananas
2 cups of Wholemeal, Self Raising Flour
¼ cup maple syrup
¼ cup pureed apple sauce
2 lightly beaten eggs
1 teaspoon vanilla extract
¼ cup melted butter

Instructions

Preheat oven to 180 degrees Celsius (or 350 degrees Fahrenheit)
Grease muffin pans or loaf pan with a bit of butter
In a large bowl, mash bananas. Add remaining ingredients and mix with a hand blender (or whisk) for 1 minute.
Spoon into muffin pans or loaf pan.

Loaf Pan: bake for 50-60min or until golden brown and springs back when you press down on top
Muffin Pan: bake for 15-20 min or until golden brown on top.

Remove from oven and allow to cool before removing from pan.

****

No Lumps Apple & Cinnamon Muffins.

Makes 12.

Texture of food is extremely important to children. My kids happily munch through sliced, diced and pureed apples, but when I cook them up in a muffin, they don't go down so well. This is my solution to my apple lumps dilemma. This is a simple, fast Muffin Recipe that can be doubled and frozen easily. Great to add to school lunches or an 'on the go' breakfast or snack.

Ingredients

1 and 1/2 cups Wholemeal Self Raising Flour
1/4 cup of melted butter. I use Organic butter.
2 Free Range Eggs
1 Teaspoon of real vanilla extract (this is optional, I just like the vanilla taste)
1/4 cup of maple syrup
1 cup of apple sauce
1 teaspoon of cinnamon (Optional 1/4 cup of chopped walnuts – for crunch

Instructions

Preheat oven to 180 degrees Celsius (or 350 degrees Fahrenheit)
Mix all ingredients together until just combined.
Spoon into greased muffin tray and bake for around 10-15 min or until golden brown on top and firm to touch. Makes 12 large or 24 small muffins.

How to Freeze & Thaw: Freshly baked muffins need to cool completely before freezing. Pack into Zip lock bags and pop into freezer. When you are ready to use, take frozen muffins out of freezer and allow thaw at room temperature for 5-8min.

****

Carrot Cake

Serves 8 - 12

Carrot Cake is a dense, moist cake that is quite rich. It does have a full cup of maple syrup, so I would consider it more of a treat than an anytime snack. If I am in a hurry, I use a 12 hole muffin tray rather than one large baking tin to reduce baking time.

Ingredients

Cake Ingredients:
2 cups grated carrots
3 eggs lightly beaten
2 teaspoons vanilla extract
1 teaspoon ground cinnamon
½ teaspoon nutmeg
2 cup wholemeal self raising flour
½ cup butter melted
¾ cup organic maple syrup or honey
½ cup chopped walnuts

Frosting ingredients:
1 cup of creamed cheese
2 teaspoon grated lemon rind
¼ cup maple syrup

Instructions
Preheat your oven to 160 degrees Celsius (or 320 degrees Fahrenheit). Combine all cake ingredients (NOT FROSTING INGREDIENTS) in a large mixing bowl Mix well until combined. Pour into a prepared 20 cm baking tin. Bake for 1 – 1½ hours or until cooked through. (15 - 20 minutes if you are using a 12 hole muffin tray). Remove from the oven and cool completely in the tin then turn out.

Frosting Instructions: Blend all three ingredients together. Spread on top of carrot cake once it has cooled to room temperature. Keeps in the fridge for up to 5 days and it freezes well too!
******

Granola bars (or Breakfast Granola if you break it up)

Makes 12 bars.

You may have most of these ingredients already in your pantry. These delicious snacks are SO easy to make that even the kids (or dad) can make them. I make these regularly as they are perfect for kid's lunches and mum (with a hot cup of tea. Ahhh Bliss).

Ingredients:
   1/2 cup flour (I use wholemeal, but almond flour works well too. Use Self Raising or add 1/4tsp baking powder if you want them to rise slightly, otherwise plain for a flatter, crunchier bar)
   1/4 cup melted butter
   1/4 cup honey
   1/4 cup peanuts or other nuts
   1/2 cup shredded coconut
   1 cup oats

Instructions
   Preheat oven to around 180 degrees Celsius (or 350 degrees Fahrenheit)
   Mix all ingredients together.
   Place in greased or baking paper lined tray.
   Press down flat (around 1-2 cm thickness is good).
   Bake for around 15-20 min until slightly brown in top.
   Take out if oven and cut into squares while hot. Muesli bars will get crispy on cooling.

*****

Easy Peanut Butter Biscuits

Makes 24 biscuits

High in protein and delicious too. Kids of all ages can make these biscuits. It's a bit like yummy play dough.

Ingredients
1 ½ cups Plain Wholemeal Flour
1 teaspoon Vanilla Extract
1 teaspoon baking soda
125g butter softened
¾ cup honey OR maple syrup
1 egg
½ cup Peanut Butter (100% peanuts)

Instructions

Preheat oven to 180 degrees Celsius (or 350 degrees Fahrenheit)
Line two baking trays with non stick paper.
Mix all ingredients together to form a sticky dough.
Shape dough into walnut sized balls and place on tray. Flatten each ball with a fork (or your fingers)
Bake for 12 – 15 min. If they are still a bit soft, turn off oven and leave biscuits inside for a couple of minutes.

****

Quick Cheese "Quackers"

Makes 24.

My little ones were never able to pronounce the word 'Cracker' correctly, so the name stuck; plus it reminds me of babies and warms my heart. So, the name is a keeper! Cheese Quakers are a lovely savoury biscuit to serve with dips or sliced veggies in school lunch boxes.

Ingredients

1 cup whole-wheat flour
100g (around 5 tablespoons of softened butter)
1 cup grated cheddar cheese
½ cup grated Parmesan cheese
Sesame seeds (OPTIONAL)

Instructions

Preheat oven to 180 degrees Celsius (or 350 degrees Fahrenheit)
Combine all ingredients and knead into a dough. If you have a food processor, then go ahead, now is the time to use it. I don't, so I opt for good old fashioned kneading.
Roll the ball into a log about 4cm / 1 ½" in diameter and place in fridge for about 15min to harden the dough to make it easier to cut. Cut with a sharp knife slice ½ cm (1/4") thick pieces off the log and place each one flat on a baking sheet.
Sprinkle half the crackers with sesame seeds (adds a bit of variety to the batch). Take a fork and gently mash down the top of each one before baking to give it fancy little lines on top.
Bake for 8 - 14 minutes or until golden brown. The thicker the crackers, the longer it will take. They will crisp on cooling.

Note from Carey: It is easy to change these crackers up a bit. We sometimes add finely chopped chives to your dough for a 'Cheese and chives' cracker.

****

Simply Yum Chocolate Biscuits

Makes 24 biscuits

I don't know what to say about these little guys. They are so quick to make and taste amazing. Get ready for Monday morning school lunches and pop these 'bikkies' in the oven whilst you are making dinner, or even better, get the kids to whip up a batch on Sunday afternoon.

Ingredients

1 ½ cups Plain Wholemeal Flour
1 teaspoon baking soda
125g butter softened
¾ cup honey OR maple syrup
1 egg
2 ½ tablespoons cocoa powder

Instructions

Preheat oven to 180 degrees Celsius (or 350 degrees Fahrenheit)
Line two baking trays with non stick paper.
Mix all ingredients together to form a sticky dough.
Shape dough into walnut sized balls and place on tray. Flatten each ball with a fork (or your fingers)
Bake for 12 – 15 min. If they are still a bit soft, turn off oven and leave biscuits inside for a couple of minutes.

****

Movie Popcorn - Three Ways

Makes a bucket full. Serves 2-4 depending on how long the Movie is.

Popcorn is the most underrated snack. It is wholegrain and easy to make. Here is the recipe for standard movie night popcorn PLUS two other quick variations to the handy snack.

Movie Popcorn Ingredients
1/2 cup popcorn
2 tablespoons oil/butter

Instructions

In a popcorn maker: Add popcorn and oil and turn on (I like this method the most :) Turn off when popping corn slows down.

In a pot on the stove: Add popcorn and oil to large pot. PUT THE LID ON (My daughter learned this one the hard way). Heat pot on stove at med - high heat. Shake the pan around a bit to make sure the kernels don't burn. Remove from heat when the popping corn slows down.

1. Either stick to the Movie Popcorn above or CHOOSE ONE of These Flavors for a bit of a change
2. Parmesan & Dried Rosemary - Shake some Parmesan and dried Rosemary for Italian style popcorn
3. Savoury - Sprinkle with Smoked Paprika for a smoky, BBQ taste

****

Tapas

Feed a Crowd.

I first stumbled upon the word 'Tapas' in Australia, yet it is a Spanish term for appetizers or snacks. Us Moms would call it vegetables and dip, but I think the word 'Tapas' makes it appear like we tried a bit harder. This is a perfect dish to take to a party or to serve on those hot afternoons when you just don't feel like a cooked dinner.

Ingredients
Variety of Vegetables sliced into 'sticks' for dipping: Celery, cucumber, carrots, red or green peppers, green beans.
Cherry tomatoes
Cheeses
Flat bread or toasted wholemeal wraps

Trio of Dips
Tzatziki
Salsa
Mango Salsa

Serve sliced vegetables, cheese and bread on a large platter with dips on the side.

****

6 Oh So Yummy Treats and Sweets

Last Minute Apple Crumble
Crepes with caramelised banana and cinnamon
Chocolate Coconut Milk Ice Cream
Chocolate Milkshake
Crunchy Caramel Corn
Fruit Popsicles three ways

Last Minute Apple Crumble

Serves 6

Apple Crumble topped with a dollop of whipped cream is blissful. The recipe calls for canned apple, so I usually have a couple of these in my pantry ready to go. It also means that when we 'feel like dessert', these ingredients are always on hand.

Ingredients

Filling
2 x 400g cans of apple (in natural juice)
½ cup maple syrup (heated)
¼ cup lemon juice (1 lemon juiced with seeds removed)
1 teaspoon cinnamon

Crumble:
½ cup finely shredded coconut
1½ cup wholemeal flour
100g butter softened
½ cup maple syrup OR honey

Instructions:

Preheat oven to 180 degrees Celsius (or 350 degrees Fahrenheit)
Prepare Filling: In a large, oven proof dish, mix together apple pieces, maple syrup, lemon juice and cinnamon.
Crumble: In a mixing bowl, add flour, coconut, butter and maple syrup until well mixed and resembles 'clumpy crumbs'.
Spread crumble on top of apple mixture. Bake for around ½ an hour or until top is a golden brown.
Serve with whipped cream.

****

Crepes with caramelized banana, cinnamon, lemon & maple syrup

Makes 6 crepes.

OK, so this may be in the dessert section, but feel free to have this for breakfast too. For a more savoury breakfast option, you can skip the maple syrup and fill your crepe with bacon and egg instead.

Ingredients

Crepes
2 large whole eggs
1/2 cup milk
1 cup whole wheat flour
1 tbsp melted butter

Filling:
2 Bananas (sliced long ways down the middle and lightly fried until heated through and golden brown on outside)
Cinnamon
½ lemon
¼ cup heated maple syrup

Instructions

In a large mixing bowl, whisk together everything until smooth. Set aside for around 15 minutes.
To prevent sticking, oil your pan with a wipe of butter.
With a soup spoon, ladle about 4 tablespoons of batter into your oiled pan.
Rotate the pan to get the batter to spread thinly and evenly over the base of the pan. Try to get your crepe to spread as thinly as possible. Cook on low to medium heat, flip once bubbles start to form on your crepe. Cooked side will be golden brown. Watch your heat. It needs to stay on medium.

To Serve: Wrap crepe around a slice of banana. Sprinkle with cinnamon and squeeze of lemon. Pour hot maple syrup on top and serve to happy children! These crepes are very versatile. I don't sweeten them so they can be used as savory wraps in school lunches too.

****

Chocolate Coconut Milk Ice Cream

Serves 4.

This ice cream tastes as if it were made in a deluxe ice cream parlor in the fancy part of town. It is rich and creamy and once you try it, you will not go back. I am confident that it's that good!

Ingredients:

3 cups of coconut milk (about two cans)
2/3 cup of cocoa powder
1/2 cup pure maple syrup
1 teaspoon vanilla extract

Instructions:

Whisk cocoa powder in a small amount of coconut milk, until smooth. Add the rest of the ingredients and whisk until well combined OR pop all ingredients in blender for a couple seconds until smooth. Place in freezer friendly tub (I use a lunch box) and place in freezer.

Note on Freezing: The ice cream does set very hard. I normally take it out about 5 minutes before serving to soften it up a bit.

*****

Chocolate Milkshake

Makes two servings, so increase ingredients according to number of servings needed. We like our milkshake served COLD as makes it feel a bit more like a treat. I freeze the banana and the Greek yogurt before making the milkshake. It is well worth the effort!

Ingredients

1 frozen banana (then peeled and cut into slices)
1/2 cup of frozen Greek yogurt (approx 4 ice cubes)
1 Tablespoon cocoa powder
1/2 cup coconut milk
2 teaspoons honey or maple syrup (add more of less to taste)

Instructions

Add all ingredients to blender and blend on high until combined and milk shake consistency is achieved.

****

Caramel Corn

Serves 4

This is a perfect treat to make for a kids birthday party. I serve it up in individual party bags and kids love it.

Ingredients
  4 cups air popped corn
  1/4 cup butter
  1/4 cup honey

Popcorn Instructions
In a popcorn maker: Add popcorn and oil and turn on (I like this method the most :) Turn off when popping corn slows down.

In a pot on the stove: Add popcorn and oil to large pot. PUT THE LID ON. Heat on stove at med - high heat. Shake the pan around a bit to make sure the kernels don't burn. Remove from heat when the popping corn slows down.

Caramel Instructions
Heat butter and honey in a pot. Bring to the boil and then allow to simmer for approx 5 minutes. STIR THE ENTIRE TIME. Caramel with thicken and darken slightly.
Pour caramel over popped corn and stir through.

Please note: Caramel is SUPER NOT. Use a spoon not your hands. Allow to cool and serve.

*****

Fruit Popsicles three ways

All of these recipes make around 6 to 10 ice blocks, but this will depend on the size of your mould. These colourful, fruity ice blocks are easy to whip up and store in the freezer. Be adventurous and feel free to replace fruit with your child's favourites.

Strawberry and yogurt
    1 punnet strawberries, washed with stems removed
    1 cup (250 ml) water / coconut water
    1 cup (250 ml) natural yoghurt

Banana & coconut
    2 ripe bananas
    1 can of coconut milk
    1 cup water
    ½ cup finely shredded coconut (optional)
    1 teaspoon vanilla extract

Banana, Mango and Pineapple
    2 ripe mangoes, skinned and chopped – about 1 cup. (You can use canned mango in natural juices if you don't have mangoes nearby)
    1 banana
    1 cup fresh or canned pineapple chunks
    1/2 cup water or coconut water

Instructions (for all three)
Blend all ingredients until smooth. Pour into ice block moulds and freeze overnight. Ice Pop Tip: to remove ice blocks from moulds, run it quickly under warm water. The ice blocks will then slide out from mould easily.

****

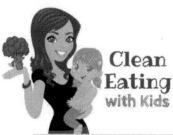

Clean Eating with Kids

CLEAN EATING
SHOPPING LIST
Real Food for Real Families.

Meat / Protein
- ☐ Eggs
- ☐ Beef – Minced / Roast
- ☐ Chicken – Pieces or Whole
- ☐ Bacon (Free Range)
- ☐ Tuna (canned or fresh)
- ☐ Salmon (Canned or fresh)
- ☐ Fish (All types sustainably caught)

Sweeteners
- ☐ Apple Sauce
- ☐ Honey
- ☐ Maple Syrup

Fruit
- ☐ Bananas
- ☐ Strawberries
- ☐ Watermelon
- ☐ Melon
- ☐ Kiwi Fruit
- ☐ Grapes
- ☐ Lemon or limes
- ☐ Pineapple (fresh or canned)
- ☐ Apple (canned, pureed, fresh)

Whole wheat / Cereals/ Grains and Pasta
- ☐ Wholemeal Plain Flour
- ☐ Wholemeal Self Raising Flour
- ☐ Oats
- ☐ Natural Muesli
- ☐ Wholewheat Pasta (all types)
- ☐ Wholegrain graps
- ☐ Cous Cous
- ☐ Basmati rice

Dairy and Substitutes
- ☐ Sour Cream
- ☐ Cottage Cheese
- ☐ Butter
- ☐ Milk
- ☐ Greek Yogurt
- ☐ Almond Milk
- ☐ Cheese
- ☐ Parmesan Cheese
- ☐ Cream
- ☐ Cream cheese
- ☐ Coconut milk / Cream

Vegetables / fruit
- ☐ Zucchini
- ☐ Mushrooms
- ☐ Onions
- ☐ Lettuce
- ☐ Carrots
- ☐ Sweet potato
- ☐ Corn (fresh or frozen)
- ☐ Spring Onion
- ☐ Cabbage
- ☐ Pumpkin
- ☐ Potatoes
- ☐ Capsicum
- ☐ Cucumber
- ☐ Celery
- ☐ Tomato (fresh or canned)
- ☐ Leeks
- ☐ Peas (fresh or frozen)
- ☐ Beans (fresh or frozen)
- ☐ Beetroot (fresh or canned)
- ☐ Avocadoes
- ☐ Spinach
- ☐ Cauliflower

Herbs & Spices
- ☐ Garlic
- ☐ Parsley
- ☐ Chives
- ☐ Coriander
- ☐ Mint
- ☐ Olive Oil or other
- ☐ Black Pepper
- ☐ Sea Salt
- ☐ Rosemary
- ☐ Onion Powder
- ☐ Thyme
- ☐ Ground Ginger
- ☐ Garam Masala
- ☐ Tumeric

Seeds / Nuts
- ☐ Pine Nuts
- ☐ Cashews
- ☐ Almonds
- ☐ Peanuts
- ☐ Coconut (shredded)
- ☐ Raisins
- ☐ Sesame Seeds

Drinks
- ☐ WATER
- ☐ Water and more
- ☐ Water

Pantry Items
- ☐ Natural Peanut Butter
- ☐ Clean Mayonnaise
- ☐ Olive oil
- ☐ Organic Pasta Sauce (bottled)
- ☐ Organic Tomato Sauce
- ☐ Dijon Mustard
- ☐ Vanilla Extract
- ☐ Stock – Chicken / Vegetable
- ☐ Cocoa Powder

www.cleaneatingwithkids.com

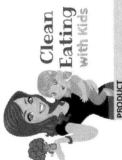

CLEAN EATING FREEZER CHART

How long will it keep? A Quick Reference Guide to Freezing Real Food.

These times assume that the freezer temperature is maintained at 0°F (-18°C) or colder. The storage time is for quality only. Frozen foods remain safe well past these dates. NOTE: When freezing liquids, allow space in the container for expansion.

Clean Eating with Kids

PRODUCT	MONTHS IN FREEZER
CHEESE (Except those listed below)	6 to 9
Cottage Cheese, cream cheese, feta, goats cheese, fresh mozzarella, Parmesan	Not Recommended
DAIRY PRODUCTS	
Butter	6 to 9
Cream	4
Ice Cream	1 to 2
Milk	3
Yogurt	1 to 2
FISH & SEAFOOD	
Clams, mussels, oysters, shrimp, scallops	3 to 6
Fatty fish (salmon, bluefin, mackerel, perch)	2 to 3
Lean Fish (flounder, haddock, sole)	6
FRESH FRUIT (PREPARED FOR FREEZING)	
All fruit except those listed below	10 to 12
Avocadoes, Bananas	3
Citrus Fruit	4 to 6
Juices	8 to 12
POULTRY	
Uncooked Poultry Whole	4
Uncooked Poultry Pieces	9
Cooked Poultry All	4

PRODUCT	MONTHS IN FREEZER
FRESH VEGETABLES (PREPARED FOR FREEZING)	
Artichokes, Eggplant	6 to 8
Asparagus, turnips	8 to 10
Beens, beets, bok choy, broccoli, brussel sprouts, carrots, cauliflower, corn, greens, leeks, mushrooms, onions, peas, peppers, spinach, squash	10 to 12
Bamboo Shoots, cabbage, celery, cucumbers, salad greens, watercress	Not recommended
MEAT / POULTRY	
Cooked	2 to 3
Ham & Lunch meats	1 to 2
Bacon / Sausage	1 to 2
Uncooked /Ground	3 to 4
Uncooked roasts, steaks, chops	4 to 12
Uncooked Wild Game	8 to 12
MISCELLANEOUS	
Cakes	4 to 6
Casseroles	2 to 3
Cookie dough	2
Cookies	3
Fruit pies baked	2 to 4
Fruit pies unbaked	8
Pastry unbaked	2
Soups and Stews	2 to 3
Yeast breads	6
Yeast dough	2 weeks

Adapted from Food Safety and Inspection Services

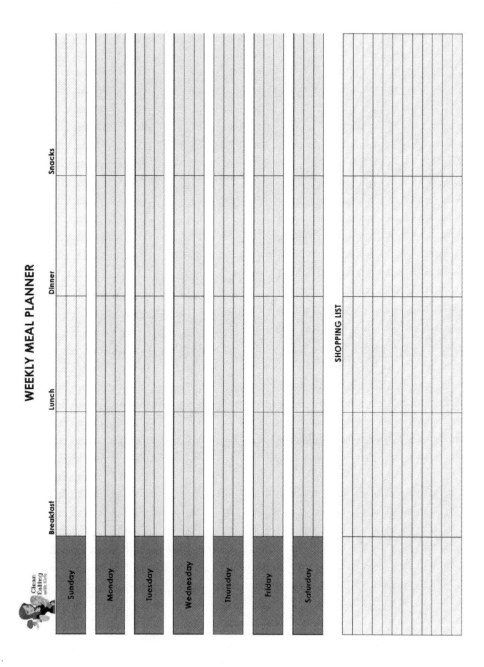

WEEKLY MEAL PLANNER

	Breakfast	Lunch	Dinner	Snacks
Sunday				
Monday				
Tuesday				
Wednesday				
Thursday				
Friday				
Saturday				

SHOPPING LIST

FURTHER READING & REFERENCES

"Clean Eating for Dummies", Wiley Publishing Inc. 2011

"Meatless Monday" © 2003 - 2014 The Monday Campaigns, Inc
www.meatlessmonday.com/about-us/why-meatless/

Sugar vs Cocaine Study 2007
http://www.ncbi.nlm.nih.gov/pmc/articles/PMC1931610/

Feeding the brain, Dr Keith Conners

Facts on Obesity and the effects on our Children.
http://www.cdc.gov/healthyyouth/obesity/facts.htm

1. The Omnivores Dilemma: A Natural History of Four Meals, 2007, Michael Pollan.

Go to www.cleaneatingwithkids.com/resources for some excellent websites that I use to find more clean eating recipes to try at home (I have added this as a link because I add to this list all the time and it's easier to update on my website as these resources change).

And of course, please stop by and visit my website anytime at www.cleaneatingwithkids.com and sign up for my Newsletter for loads more information on clean eating with kids – sent right to your inbox.

ABOUT THE AUTHOR

Carey lives in sunny Queensland, Australia with her husband, four kids, 2 dogs, 2 cats, 2 chickens and 6 guinea pigs (but that's a whole other story).

You can connect with her on her website or Facebook page.

www.cleaneatingwithkids.com
www.facebook.com/cleaneatingwithkids

One Last Thing ....

You can connect with me on my
website, www.cleaneatingwithkids.com
Facebook Page www.Facebook.com/cleaneatingwithkids or
send me an email at cleaneatingwithkids@gmail.com.

I would love to hear how your journey with Clean Eating is
going.

xxo
Carey

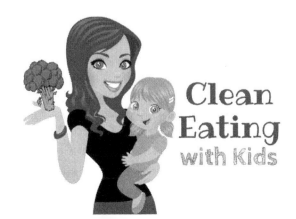

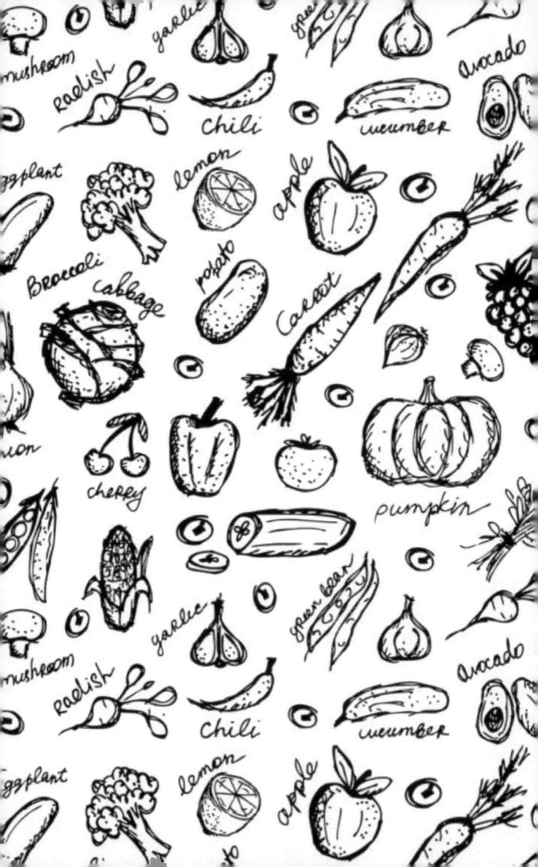

Made in the USA
Columbia, SC
02 November 2020